A Patient's Survival Guide

or

Never Get Naked . . .
On Your First Visit!

WE THINK IT'S GREAT!

"In nearly 30 years ...I have not seen a publication which provides more useful, basic information. [Helps patient] get quality care and [helps] employer contain costs...a great book."

R. A., Executive Vice President
Insurance Claims Payer

"...Put concepts to work...saved 2 hours of my time, a $45 office visit and no more side effects."

G. C., Patient

"Our claim loss ratio was over 115%...reduced to less than 50% and employees perceived [it] as an employee benefit".

K. D., Personnel Director
Real Estate Development Company

"...I have found the contents so informative and useful. [It is my] primary resource material."

W. M., Major Accounts Consultant
Major Insurance Company

Published by Med. Ed.

All inquiries should be addressed to: Reorder from:

    Med. Ed. Inc.   Med. Ed. Inc.
    P.O. Box 40696   P.O. Box 40696
    Mesa, Arizona 85274-0696   Mesa, Arizona 85274-0696

Library of Congress Cataloging-in-Publication Data
Ellig, David H.
    A Patient's Survival Guide, or, Never Get Naked On Your First Visit.

    p. cm.
    Includes index.
    ISBN 0-9628311-0-7

1.   Medicine, Popular.
2.   Consumer protection.
3.   Self-care, Health.
4.   Medical care--Citizen participation.
I.   Title

RC81.E46 1991   91-34795
362.1--dc20

WARNING

Notice: The information in this book is true and complete to the best of our knowledge. This book is intended only as an informative guide for those wishing to know more about their medical treatment options. In no way is this book intended to replace, countermand or conflict with the advice given to you by your doctor.

There are many variables to any illness or surgical condition. Your doctor knows your symptoms, signs, allergies, general health and the many other variables that challenge his/her judgment in caring for you as a patient.

The ultimate decision concerning any surgery or treatment should be made between you and your doctor, and we strongly recommend that you follow his/her advice. The information in this book is general and is offered with no guarantees on the part of the authors or Med. Ed., Inc. The authors and publisher disclaim all liability in connection with the use of this book.

Published by Med. Ed., Inc.
Med. Ed. Publishing
P.O. Box 40696
Mesa, AZ 85274
(602) 345-1943

ISBN: 0-9628311-0-7
Library of Congress Catalog Card
Number 90-92333
©1991 D. H. Ellig
Printed in U.S.A.
1st Printing

Other Books By D. H. Ellig:
    Stimulating Questions for Doctors, Hospitals, Labs © 1988
    Patient's Handbook © 1988
    Going To The Hospital? © 1988

DEDICATION
To All Future Patients

Most of us are fortunate to enter the healthcare delivery system for major surgery only once or twice in our lives. The problem with this good luck is that when we enter the healthcare delivery system for the first time we are inexperienced neophytes, interacting with professionals who provide this unique service as a day in and day out job.

Since it is our first experience we don't know what to expect, how to react, or how to interact with our care givers. We are, therefore, at a disadvantage and may not raise questions which are totally appropriate and which can affect our healthcare outcomes.

This book will provide the first-time patient the benefit of the experiences of many prior patient visits so the patient can receive the best quality of healthcare at the best price for treatment outcomes that are understood.

There is much good in the healthcare system, some bad. The ideas and concepts in this book may help you avoid some of the bad. It is not possible to avoid all the bad because healthcare providers are human and mistakes will be made. What you want to avoid is those providers who are not qualified or who make more mistakes than average or place us at unnecessary risk by recommending unnecessary surgery.

WE THINK IT'S GREAT, TOO!

"The concept is blatantly needed by employees and your booklet, newsletter, promo pieces are dynamite! It can only be a WINNER and I'm proud to have been apart of your audience selected to critique this masterpiece!"

J. P., Health Promotion Consultant

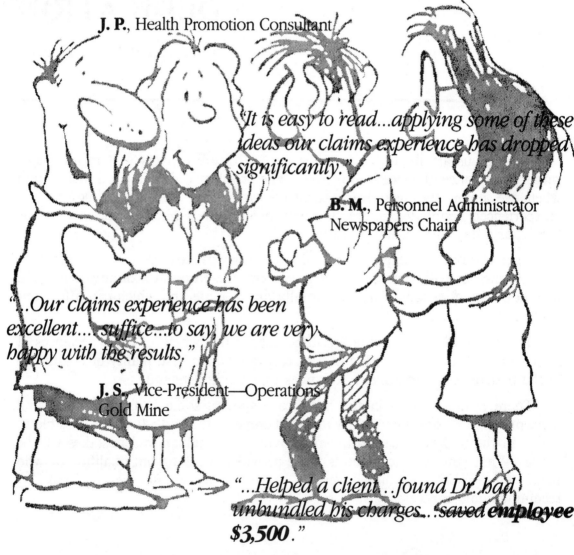

"It is easy to read...applying some of these ideas our claims experience has dropped significantly."

B. M., Personnel Administrator
Newspapers Chain

"...Our claims experience has been excellent... suffice...to say, we are very happy with the results."

J. S., Vice-President—Operations
Gold Mine

*"...Helped a client...found Dr. had unbundled his charges...saved **employee $3,500**."*

G. C., Benefits Consultant

PREFACE

This book was originally conceived as a tool to address the issue of healthcare costs for the author's corporate clients and their employees. Applying the ideas presented in this book will affect the cost of medical treatment, but the real issue is the quality of care offered by the medical profession, and the lack of information given to patients. When a much smaller version of this book (which contained only questions) was distributed to employees, it was quickly discovered that the healthcare cost issue was not solely one of cost, but also an issue of the lack of consumer information. We found that the patient was provided with very little quality or price information with which to make an informed buying decision. We decided that what was needed was not only a book of questions, but a book with answers and referral sources where answers could be found.

As a result of this small experiment to provide information to patients, we found that people really want to be involved and informed about their medical care. We also found that people could understand complex medical treatment plans when given the right information. Some employees even found that their new knowledge allowed them to be a better judge of the quality of a proposed healthcare provider. Sometimes they found they knew more than the healthcare provider and, as a result, didn't feel comfortable with that healthcare provider.

This was a surprising finding, since the prevailing attitude in the healthcare and insurance industry is that the patient doesn't care or isn't capable of understanding his treatment program.

This book encourages an open doctor/patient dialogue. We found some healthcare providers were reluctant to participate in this open dialogue process or challenged the need for patient involvement. The employees easily resolved this issue by simply going to another healthcare provider.

The employers who were involved in the development of the concepts of this book were rewarded with lower medical cost and a new employee benefit. The employees came to realize that healthcare treatment is expensive and that they should and can get the best quality care for the money spent.

ACKNOWLEDGEMENTS

I want to thank all of the people who have helped to get this book published.

For motivation — I'd like to thank all of my clients, their employees and other patients who encouraged and motivated me to write this book and provided their healthcare experiences.

For guidance — I would like to thank all of the professionals who provided insight and review. These people provided a tremendous amount of help and credibility to the book. Many professionals recognize the problems in the industry but cannot publicly speak out due to fear of censure and possible loss of employment. A partial list of the contributors: healthcare providers, professionals and administrators; TPA (third party administrators) and their staff; benefit consultants and insurance brokers, insurance company marketing personnel, nurses, medical malpractice attorney, medical malpractice broker and Utilization Review firms, search analysts and financial planners.

For help — I want to thank all of the proofreaders, editors, layout personnel, printers, authors, librarians, Joe Gunsten the illustrator, and Bob McCarroll and his staff for the cover layout. And finally Diane Ruopsa of Paper Chase who has spent many hours typing these 70,000 words at least 14 times and has become a "smart" medical consumer. Thank you all very much.

Quick Reference

Never Get Naked...On Your First Visit

TABLE OF CONTENTS

Never Get Naked...On Your First Visit

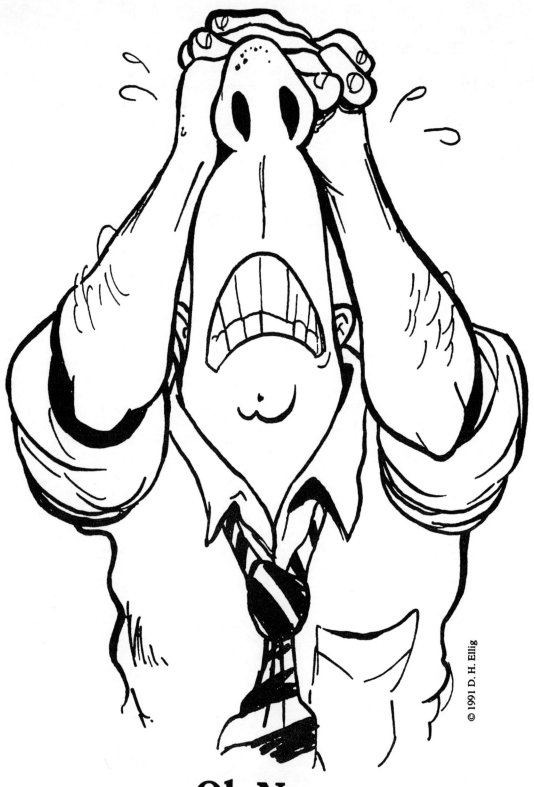

© 1991 D. H. Ellig

Oh No....

xx

INTRODUCTION

Have you ever left the doctor's office and thought,

Oh, I wish I would have asked about . . . or

I forgot to tell the doctor about . . . or

I wonder if I was told everything . . .

or three months later said . . .

If I only knew then what I know now, I would have . . . or

Holy moly! That was expensive, I owe $$$!!!

(I wonder if they would take my first born as a down payment?)

Many people in the healthcare industry express the opinion that patients don't want to be involved with their care or are not smart enough to be involved with their care. *This is not true!* The problem is that for many patients it is the first time they have had major medical treatment and don't know what or how to ask questions or where to get treatment information in a language they can understand. Also, most patients are not given adequate information necessary to make an informed decision. This book provides the patient access to a base of knowledge and sources so that even the first-time patient can act like a veteran who has survived numerous encounters with the healthcare industry.

The material in this book is compiled from the experiences of many patient visits and is designed to help you be at ease after a visit to a healthcare provider because you are fully informed or know where to get the answers.

If the ideas in this book are applied, you won't be surprised, you won't be intimidated; you'll get better care and your treatment outcomes will be better, because you will be an involved patient fully coordinating your care with your healthcare provider.

Many times patients are not involved in their treatment; they are simply a body being repaired. We believe the lack of active patient involvement with their care is due, in a large part, to intimidation as a result of four factors:

fear,
they don't know *what questions to ask*
they don't know they have a *right to ask questions*
they don't know *questions must be answered*

Many patients are easily intimidated by healthcare providers because the combination of lack of knowledge, fear and the presence of all-powerful figures who know all the answers. Hopefully, this book will provide information which will lessen the intimidation and make patients more at ease with their treatment and healthcare providers.

Fear

Many patients cannot or do not become involved with their care because of fear — fear of the unknown and concern for one's life. The fear places patients in an emotional state where they only want results — to be cured. This book will help resolve some of the fear of the unknown, since it provides methods to get answers about your condition and information sources you can access to obtain almost as much information as the healthcare provider. Questions have been formatted to help the patient formulate important questions about treatment.

Don't Know What Questions to Ask

This book provides important questions for patients to ask healthcare providers about their treatment plans and the healthcare provider's experience. The list of questions is quite extensive and provides reasons why the questions are important. This book should be considered only the starting point. Every patient will have more questions than could possibly be listed, because of his individual condition, needs and concerns. At the very least, the book is a starting point for an open doctor/patient dialogue.

The Right to Ask and the Obligation to Answer

Surprisingly many patients don't know they have a legal right to ask questions and the doctor has a legal, ethical and moral obligation to answer questions honestly. The chapter on informed consent discusses this doctrine and what information **must** be provided the patient. If patients will ask questions, they will be answered. If a patient feels uncomfortable about asking questions of his healthcare provider, the book contains references to many other sources where answers can be obtained.

The book is organized to provide the individual patient with a step-by-step process for seeking and receiving medical treatment. The chapters are arranged to offer assistance from the time you are feeling ill, until you are out of the hospital and wondering where all the costs came from.

The book has many forms which can serve as reminders and as a source to record important healthcare issues, such as quality of care, cost and treatment risk assessment, which will help the patient to be a truly informed buyer of medical services.

What to Expect

The application of suggestions in this book will change your buying habits and will make you an unusual consumer in the healthcare industry. As such, you may experience difficulties getting providers and their staffs to respond to your questions and concerns. You will have to be persistent and maybe more diligent in your search for a provider with whom you feel comfortable.

We have also found that it takes a number of visits before you feel comfortable applying the concepts of this book. The usual experience is that the patient will not change his buying habits on the first visit, but will experience an issue addressed in the book and know that it would have been treated differently if he had applied some of the concepts suggested. This experience will give encouragement to change future buying habits on subsequent visits.

The best advice we can provide is: **never get naked on your first visit**. You have a moral obligation to yourself and your loved ones to thoroughly research the healthcare provider's qualifications, suggested treatment plan and cost before you submit to treatment.

Actually it is okay to disrobe for diagnostic purposes if you have qualified the doctor and the labs. But never get naked at the hospital until you have qualified *all* the doctors, the hospital, labs and thoroughly understand your treatment, its risks and the available alternatives.

Will It Work?

Only for the persistent patient who wants to be involved and takes an interest in their treatment. Studies show that patient information and education can positively affect outcomes. Consider the following results when patients were educated and involved.

1) 25.8 percent fewer hysterectomies
2) 33 percent fewer hospital admittances for asthmatics
3) Hypertensive and diabetic patients had lower readings
4) 60 percent fewer prostate surgeries
5) 15 percent drug cost reduction.

It is time to change the way we accept medical treatment, from one of "blind faith" in our healthcare providers to one where we can "peek" by getting more information. We need the *strength* to say "no, whoa, wait a minute, I need more information!"

Super Patient

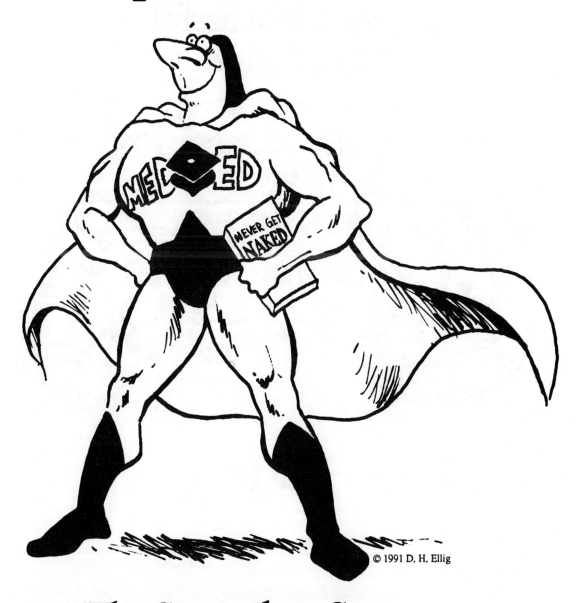

© 1991 D, H, Ellig

"The Strength to Say… No, Whoa, Wait a Minute I Need More Information"

Here's A Wonderful Little Gadget

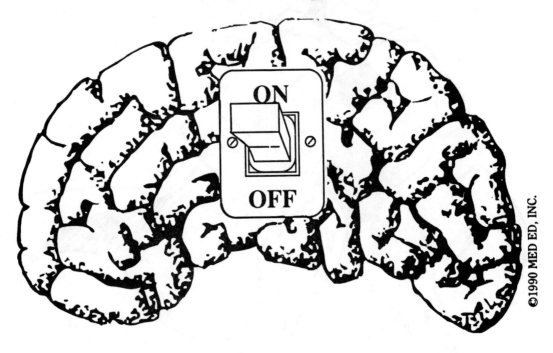

Use It!

A HEALTHCARE CONSUMER'S STATEMENT OF BELIEFS

We endorse this healthcare consumer statement of beliefs knowing that it is well grounded in legal precedence, ethical guidelines and is morally correct. We expect that our healthcare givers will not ask us to violate any of these principles.

1)   We recognize that we are **extremely vulnerable** when we require medical services and expect that our healthcare givers will treat us in a caring, open and honest manner.

2)   We recognize that **we hire doctors, hospitals and labs** to provide services for our most important possessions; our lives and those of our family and friends.

3)   We pay **substantial fees** for these services.

4)   We have a right to **expect services and skill levels** to be commensurate with the price of services.

5)   We have the **right to determine the quality** of the provider of our services.

6)   We recognize that medical services cannot be provided without our permission and we will not be asked to provide approval until we **fully understand** the qualifications of the provider, and the services to be provided, and our expectations agree with the providers'.

7)   We recognize that **only those services** we agree to may be provided.

8)   We recognize that by accepting this statement of beliefs we may discover some facts that we don't want to know, but would rather discover those facts **before** treatment **rather than after** treatment.

Finally we recognize that **our interest** in our medical treatment **is greater** than that of the healthcare giver; it is our life and lifestyle at risk, it is their vocation. We expect the healthcare giver to put **our interest before their own.**

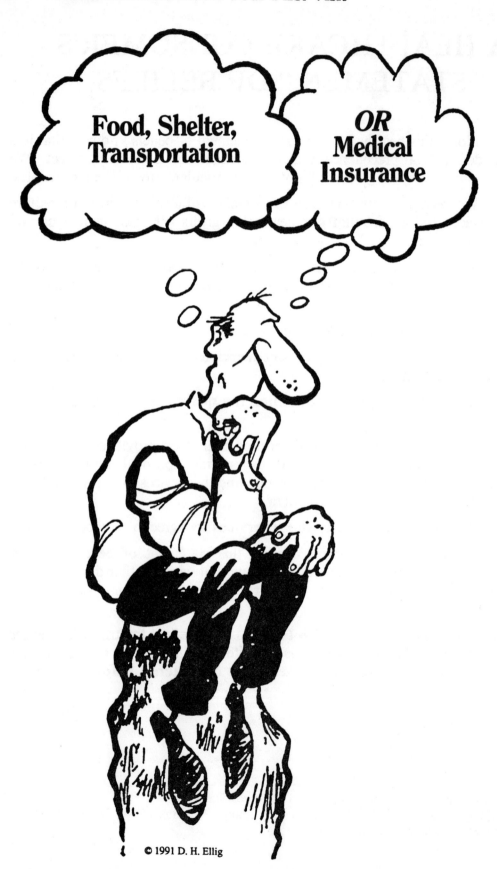

© 1991 D. H. Ellig

CHAPTER 1

NINE WORDS ABOUT COSTS

The nine words . . .

Medical insurance is **expensive** *and will become* **more** *expensive!*
(Employers will pay $22,000 per year per employee by 2000.*)

Think about the effect on wages — you'll be asked, "Do you want wages or benefits?" (Personal income rose 6 percent in 1990 — Medical insurance rose 25 percent)

The healthcare consumer has to get involved *now.*

ACTUAL INSURANCE INCREASES

Premium	Date	Years Covered
$132.20	7/1/91	5
$115.79	7/1/90	4
$103.83	7/1/89	3
$ 77.27	7/1/88	2
$ 45.56	7/1/87	1
$ 37.70	7/1/86	0

Premiums Increased 3 1/2 Times in 5 Years

* A. Foster Higgins. "Indemnity Plans: Cost, Design, Funding," 1990.

—— $92 for 7 Days in 1947 ——

STATEMENT

LAKESIDE HOSPITAL ASSOCIATION

PHONE
LINWOOD 0408

29TH AND FLORA
KANSAS CITY, MO.

ACCOUNTS PAYABLE WEEKLY
IN ADVANCE

FOR SERVICES RENDERED

ITEM	CHARGES
Room From 6-1 -47 To 6-8-47	42.00
Laboratory — Routine	6.00
Laboratory — Special	
Operating Room	20.00
Anaesthetic	20.00
Drugs and Dressings	7.00
X-Ray	
Venoclysis	
Special Nurse's Board	
Guest Meals	
Cot	
Physiotherapy	
Laundry	25
Room Service Telephone	
Newspapers	
Drug Store	
Miscellaneous	
Total	95.25
Less Payments	
Balance Due	95.25

PAID
25
6/7/47
LAKESIDE HOSPITAL
By

Estimated Deductions Of Insurance   70.00

Estimated Difference $25.25

RECEIPTS MAILED ONLY WHEN REQUESTED

$3,033 for 45 Minutes in 1991

HOSPITAL		
		N92399/F-205
		DETAIL STATEMENT

INSURANCE COMPANY	POLICY NO.	GROUP NO.	POLICYHOLDER

RESPONSIBLE PARTY		PATIENT NAME	

		ADMIT DATE	PAGE NO.
		06/26/91	3
		DISCHARGE DATE	P/T F/C DRG
		06/26/91	3 43 01
SCOTTSDALE, AZ 85261		BILL DATE	ACCT. REP.
		07/02/91	
		ACCOUNT BALANCE	
	OUT-PATIENT	3,033.30	

Please detach and return top portion with your remittance. Guarantor is responsible for any amounts due after the insurance companies make their actual payments

FOR OFFICE REFERENCE	SERVICE DATE		DESCRIPTION	QTY.	PATIENT BALANCE
		250	PHARMACY		615.60
		258	IV SOLUTIONS		131.90
		270	MED-SURG SUPPLIES		976.04
		307	LAB/UROLOGY		13.20
		360	OR SERVICES		756.26
		370	ANESTHESIA		233.70
		410	RESPIRATORY SVC		17.90
		710	RECOVERY ROOM		200.80
		730	EKG/ECC		87.90

PATIENT NAME	ACCOUNT NO.	ADMIT DATE	DISCHARGE DATE	BILL DATE	ACCOUNT REP.	
		06/26/91	06/26/91	07/02/91		3,033.30
						ACCOUNT BALANCE

DATE OF POSTING DOES NOT NECESSARILY REPRESENT THE DATE THE SERVICE WAS RENDERED.

A Home Medical Library...

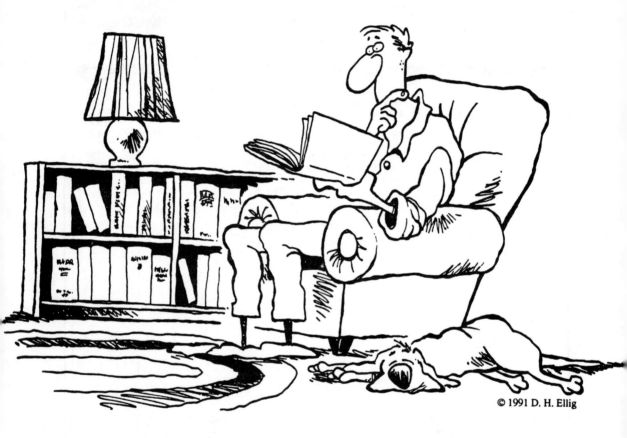

© 1991 D. H. Ellig

Is a Warm Fuzzy Feeling

CHAPTER 2

HOME MEDICAL LIBRARY

Healthcare consumers should have access to some basic medical books and newsletters that can be easily understood. A home medical library can be started for less than $25 and completely stocked for $66, less than the cost of a visit to the doctor, tests and prescriptions.

Many times we feel ill, worry about our condition or the results of the last doctor visit. The books in this chapter will provide a general understanding of many medical conditions, testing procedures and drugs. Most people are more comfortable when they have a general understanding of their illness, condition or test results from an unbiased second source. Your medical library will be a great help in understanding what your doctor said. None of the books, however, provide treatment success probabilities. For probabilities you will have to refer to medical studies as discussed in Chapter 8.

Why A Medical Library Is Important

****

CONCEPT AT WORK:

First Story — An individual started taking a new drug and each morning his heart would race, almost palpitate. He was concerned about his condition and was faced with a doctor visit, quit taking the drug, or both. Then he remembered this book and the suggestion of a medical library with a book on drugs. He purchased one of the suggested drug books and discovered that a side effect of the drug was that when taken with caffeine, the heart would race. The next morning he had decaffeinated coffee and no heart palpitations. Result: for $7.00 (the price of the book) he didn't have to inconvenience his schedule with a doctor visit, pay for an office visit, or stop taking his medication.

Second Story — Another individual's child was being treated for a fairly serious illness. The medical library was consulted for the disease and it confirmed that, yes, the child had these symptoms, they are treated this way, the drug dosage was "x," and the child should be well in "x" weeks. A copy of the drug warnings from one of the books was given to the child so he would know the side effects, warnings and what to do if he forgot to take a pill. Result: The parent felt at ease, he and the doctor were doing the right thing.

****

The following books and newsletters have been selected because they are easy to understand and cover many common medical issues. The prices are current suggested prices and may vary. A majority of these books are also available in most libraries, but you will use these books many times and it may be worthwhile to have them at home.

BOOKS

A well stocked home medical library would include a selection of one book from each of the following categories.

Self-Care	Medical Testing
Drugs	Medical Dictionary

Self-Care

The books referred to in this section are books to help you determine when a doctor visit is appropriate, be delayed or if the condition can be treated at home.

The American Medical Association Family Medical Guide

Random House   **Recommended**
201 50th Street   Price $29.95
New York, NY 10036

Has detailed self-diagnosis flow charts and other illustrations to help consumer understand medical conditions. Provides the basics to start an open dialogue with the doctor.

Complete Guide to Symptoms, Illness and Surgery, by H. Winter Griffith, M.D.

Putnam Publishing   **Recommended**
200 Madison Ave.   Price $14.95
New York, NY 10016

This book may be more difficult to find than the others, but it is well written, easy to understand and complete. Most libraries should have it on their shelves. The book discusses common symptoms, diseases, therapies and surgical procedures, plus other self-help topics, such as diets, reducing stress and self-examinations.

Healthwise Handbook, by Donald W. Kemper, Kathleen E. McIntosh and Toni M. Roberts

Healthwise, Inc.   Price $12.95
P.O. Box 1989
Boise, ID 83701

This book discusses various symptoms and conditions, and provides instructions on how to treat them at home and when to see the doctor. It also discusses how to maintain health records, what you should have in your medicine chest, and suggests eating habits and exercise programs.

Signs & Symptoms

Nurse's Reference Library   Price $29.95
Springhouse Corporation
1111 Bethlehem Pike
Spring House, PA 19477

This book will probably be available at the library or by special order at the bookstore. It is an excellent book for finding out what is wrong with you, either before your doctor visit and after the visit. It is written in easy to read terms and is very extensive. You will find in it many other medical and physical things that you have often puzzled about.

Another book in this series is *Assessment* and may be of interest since it has patient complaint charts which reference a possible illness or condition.

Take Care of Yourself: A Consumer's Guide to Medical Care, by Donald M. Vickery, M.D., and James F. Fries, M.D.

Addison-Wesley Publishing Co.   Price $14.95
1 Jacob Way
Reading, MA 01867

This book uses a flowchart approach to decide when to see a doctor and when to use home suggested treatments. It addresses many common illnesses and conditions that occur in our lives.

Drugs

****

CONCEPT AT WORK:

You are sitting at home watching TV and a drug commercial advertising a new antihistamine available only by prescription is shown and concludes with, "See your doctor about "x." You see your doctor and he prescribes "x" at a cost of $50.00 for 30 tablets. It has now cost almost $100 ($50 for drugs and $50 for office visit).

Later you buy the *Pill Book* and look up your new improved antihistamine. Under the special information section it concludes; "equally effective antihistamines are sold without prescription and for relatively little money."

Thirty tablets of an over-the-counter antihistamine could have been purchased for $2.49.

****

Because drug manufacturers, pharmacies and physicians do a poor job of providing information in a readable format, every household should have one of these books. The typical drug label provided by the pharmacy provides the name of the drug, its strength and instructions of *how often* and *how long* to take. They may occasionally have a small warning such as "don't operate hazardous equipment" or, "may cause drowsiness."

All of the suggested books have extensive information about drugs such as:

General Information	Drug Interactions
Why Prescribed	Food Interactions
Cautions and Warnings	Usual Dosage
Pregnancy/Breast Feeding	Overdosage Treatment
Senior Cautions	Special Warnings
Possible Side Effects	Missed Dosage Information

They provide much information in a text that is easy to read and understand.

The New Consumer Drug Digest, by the American Society of Hospital
  Pharmacists

Facts on File, Inc.   Price $10.95
460 Park Avenue South
New York, NY 10016

This digest helps consumers understand the drugs they are taking, why they
are taking them, why the doctor prescribed them, the side effects and any
precautions. It also describes how patients can monitor their own drug therapy.

*The Pill Book: The Illustrated Guide to the Most Prescribed Drugs in the United
  States*

Bantam Books   **Recommended**
666 Fifth Avenue   Price $5.95
New York, NY 10103

This book has color illustrations of 1600 frequently prescribed pills showing
both generic and brand names. It also addresses cautions and warnings, possible
side effects, adverse reactions and usual dosage in easy to understand non-medical
jargon. It provides a chart of drug interactions for the consumer who is taking
more than one medication. **It has special explanations of drug effects and
warnings for seniors.**

The Essential Guide to Nonprescription Drugs, by David R. Zimmerman

Harper and Row Publisher   Price $12.95
10 East 53rd Street
New York, NY 10022

This is a guide to nonprescription drugs indexed by category of drug in
alphabetical order. It is derived from the FDA review of over-the-counter drugs.

The Essential Guide to Prescription Drugs, by James W. Long

Harper Collins Inc.   Price $14.95
10 East 53rd Street
New York, NY 10022

May be too technical in some sections but is thorough and well organized.
Has a helpful section concerning drug treatments for specific conditions and
diseases. Covers only the most frequently prescribed drugs. Also has information
on most over-the-counter drugs.

Medical Testing

The Complete Book of Medical Tests: A Lifetime Guide for You and Your Family, by Mark A. Moskowitz, M.D., and Michael E. Osband, M.D.

Fawcett Columbine   Price $17.50
201 East 50th Street
New York, NY 10022

This book provides information about tests in general, when the doctor should recommend various tests and a section on self-testing at home.

The People's Book of Medical Tests, by David S. Sobel, M.D., and Tom Ferguson, M.D.

Summit Books/Simon and Schuster, Inc.   Price $14.95
Simon and Schuster Building
1230 Avenue of the Americas
New York, NY 10020

This book provides information about many medical tests, how the procedure is performed, risks, side effects, cost and information about test results.

Complete Guide to Medical Tests, by H. Winter Griffith, M.D.

Fisher Books   **Recommended**
P.O. Box 38040   Price $19.95
Tucson, AZ 85740-8040

Medical tests are described in simple language and format is easy to follow. Book describes how tests are performed, how you'll feel and what to expect from the results. The book also provides estimated costs of the test which may be slightly outdated due to the rapid rise in medical cost.

The Patient's Guide to Medical Tests, by Pinckney and Pinckney

Facts on File, Inc.   Price $12.95
460 Park Avenue South
New York, NY 10016

Text reviews 1,000 medical tests for the medical consumer, giving consumer-oriented information about costs, risks, results and why test should be performed.

Medical Dictionary

The medical dictionary may also be an encyclopedia of medical information such as:

Definition of Terms	Diagnosis
Type of Disease	Treatment
Cause and Incidence	Outlook
Symptoms and Signs	

The American Medical Association Encyclopedia of Medicine

Random House   Price $44.95
201 E. 50th Street
New York, NY 10036

This is more than a medical dictionary. It is indexed by medical terms, symptoms, diseases, drugs and treatments. The content of its 1,110 pages covers many issues briefly, and provides basic understanding of medical terminology.

The Bantam Medical Dictionary

Bantam Books   **Recommended**
666 Fifth Avenue   Price $5.95
New York, NY 10103

A complete, easy to read medical dictionary with a fair amount of illustrations. Medical terms used in definitions are cross-referenced for ease of understanding. Its small print may be difficult for those with weak eye sight.

The Mosby Medical Encyclopedia

New American Library   Price $12.50
1633 Broadway
New York, NY 10019

This is a very complete medical dictionary. Provides signs and symptoms, information about drug interactions and other information. The book is written to provide the patient with an understanding of medical jargon.

One More Book

9,479 Questionable Doctors — Disciplined by States or the Federal Government

Public Citizen Health Research Group
2000 P Street, NW
Washington, DC 20036

Price $53.00 All U.S.
$12.00 One State

This book lists, by state, doctors who have had some type of action filed and/or were disciplined for various charges by both state and federal government agencies.

It is a good book to refer to, particularly if you are new in an area. The book provides certain qualifications and suggested cautions on its use. The book is available at public libraries in the reference section and some libraries will provide a service of researching the doctors name over the telephone.

Title changes every year, 1990 edition was *6,892 Questionable Doctors.*

Recommended Library

The library selections shown are based on experience of consumer choices. It is sequenced based on cost versus benefits (just like medical decisions should be). If you can't afford them all at one time you can purchase as needed. These books are entry level books and if you desire more technical books you may change the list.

Price	Book Title	Consumer	Employer
$ 5.95	*Pill Book*	X	X
$14.95	*A Complete Guide to Symptoms, Illness, Surgery*	X	X
$ 5.95	*Bantam Medical Dictionary*	X	X
$17.95	*Complete Guide to Medical Tests*	X	X
$29.95	*AMA Family Medical Guide*	X	X
$10.00	*Community Support Group Directory*		X
$29.95	*The Consumer Health Information Source Book*		X
$53 or $12	*9,479 Questionable Doctors*		X
$24 ea.	Two Consumer Medical Newsletters		X

NOTE: The cost of a <u>complete</u> library is less than one month's medical premium.

NEWSLETTERS AND PERIODICALS

Periodicals can be a very helpful source of the most recent data on a particular illness. There are many available dedicated to those individuals who have an ongoing illness or condition that requires continuing treatment.

Some examples of periodicals and newsletters are:

Alcoholism and Addiction - $18.75
Bimonthly
Alcom Inc.
P.O. Box 31329
Seattle, WA
The magazine discusses alcoholism and other addictions featuring articles on treatment programs, facilities and news items of interest. Book reviews are also provided.

Allergy Relief Newsletter - $30.00 Monthly
Rodale Press
33 E. Miner Street
Emmaus, PA 18049
Discusses issues regarding allergies and asthma.

Arthritis Today - Free Quarterly
Arthritis Foundation
1314 Spring Street
Atlanta, GA 30309
Discusses what's new in arthritis treatment.

Back to Health - $17.55 Monthly
Back Pain Magazine Inc.
1761 W. Hillsboro Blvd.
Deerfield Beach, FL 33442
Information about back pain treatment programs and physical fitness. Many self-care programs are addressed.

Cancer News - Free Three Per Year
American Cancer Society
3340 Peachtree Road, N.E.
Atlanta, GA 30020
Provides information about new cancer treatment programs, where research is being done and other general cancer topics.

Diabetes Self Management - $18.00
Bimonthly
P.O. Box 52890
Boulder, CO 80322
This magazine discusses diabetic conditions and provides ways of helping patients control and manage their diabetes though the use of tips, guides and procedures. Magazine also references other magazines and books.

FDA Consumer - $19.00 Ten Issues Per Year
Superintendent of Documents
U.S. Government Printing Office
Washington, DC 20402
Contains information about recent court actions by the FDA, plus many articles on health care related subject. A good newsletter to keep you updated on what's happening.

Health Facts - $18.00 Monthly
Center for Medical Consumers
237 Thompson Street
New York, NY 10012
A good publication for the health care consumer. Articles provide consumer information about effectiveness of medical methods, testing and drugs.

Health Letter - $18.00 Monthly
The Public Citizen Health Research Group
2000 P Street, NW
Washington, DC 20036
A health care consumer advocacy newsletter which is understandable since Ralph Nader is co-founder. Focuses on health care quality, cost and consumer tips.

Looking Up Times Newsletter
P.O. Box K
Augusta, ME 04332
(207) 626-3402

A newsletter dedicated to victims of sexual child abuse that discusses recovery issues and treatment.

Medical Sciences Bulletin - $19.00
Robert P. Hand
P.O. Box 186
Collegeville, PA 19426

Devoted to providing the newest information on advances in drug treatment programs.

Medical Self-Care Magazine, Inc. - $15.00
Bimonthly
P.O. Box 717
Inverness, CA 94937

Founded by a medical doctor, the magazine discusses a self-care program and review of popular medical publications.

Peoples Medical Society Newsletter - $15.00
Bimonthly
462 Walnut Street
Allentown, PA 18102

An excellent consumer advocate newsletter published by the largest consumer advocate organization. Articles are consumer-oriented. Discusses patient rights, book reviews and newest patient issues.

Prevention - $12.00 Monthly
Rodale Press
33 E. Miner Street
Emmaus, PA 18049

Probably the most well-known of the medical self-care publications.

Vegetarian Times - $19.95 Monthly
141 South Oak Park Ave.
P.O. Box 570
Oak Park, IL 60303

Of interest to vegetarians or those who would like to change their diet. Menus, diets, etc. are featured.

These newsletters and periodicals are provided as a sample of the types of *disease specific periodicals* and *newsletters* available to you.

There is a book that provides an excellent source of published material in health care for the medical consumer.

The Consumer Health Information Source Book, by Alan M. Rees/Catherine Hoffman

Oryx Press
4041 N. Central
Phoenix, AZ 85012

Provides an excellent source of published material in health care for the medical consumer. This book reviews 750 books, 75 medical newsletters and 700 pamphlets. A quick reference to this book will provide direction to many excellent detailed sources.

It can be found in the reference section of most libraries.

For those of you who would like to know what other disease specific publications are available, your library may have the following source books in their reference section:

Oxbridge Director of Newsletters

Oxbridge Communications Inc.
150 Fifth Avenue
New York, NY 10011
(212) 741-0231

This provides the same data as the standard periodical directory for all newsletters published in the United States.

The Standard Periodical Directory

Oxbridge Communications Inc.
150 Fifth Avenue
New York, NY 10011
(212) 741-0231

This book lists all periodicals published in the United States. There are 2,500 medical periodicals listed.

There are also sections on psychiatry, dentistry, health and hospitals. If you are looking for a specific illness periodical, it should be in this document. The book will tell you the publisher's name, price, phone number and address.

Ulrich International Periodicals Directory

R. R. Bowker
245 W. 17th Street
New York, NY 10011

A three volume directory of international published periodicals.

INTERESTING READING

Below are some book titles that may be available at your local library. This list is not intended to be an endorsement of the various publications, but is offered only to show the wide range of information available for your reference.

A Taste of My Own Medicine, by Dr. Edward E. Rosenbaum

Random House   Price $16.95
201 E. 50th Street
New York, NY 10022

An interesting book written by a doctor describing his experiences as a patient but only after six months of misdiagnosis by his doctor friends. He describes his shock at the way the healthcare industry treats the patient and voices his concerns.

The book was the basis for the movie "The Doctor," starring William Hurt.

A.A.R.P. Pharmacy Service Prescription Drug Handbook

American Association of Retired Persons   Price $13.95
1909 K Street N.W.
Washington, DC 20049

This handbook provides information concerning drug side effects, benefits and warnings.

The Best in Medicine: How to Get the Finest Health Care For You and Your Family, by Hubert J. Dietrich and Virginia Biddle

Harmony/Crown Publishers   Price $12.95
225 Park Avenue S.
New York, NY 10003

This book has a list of the best hospitals and clinics by medical specialty. Chapters cover transplants, cancer, cardiac care, pediatrics, etc. The list was developed from interviews with 300 doctors, medical professors and hospital administrators. They were asked where they would go for medical treatment. The book lists the facilities they selected.

Confessions of a Medical Heretic, by Robert Mendesohn

Contemporary Books   Price $3.95
180 N. Michigan Avenue
Chicago, IL 60601

Written by a physician, this book presents his opinion of questionable medical practices and treatment plans.

Dr. Dean Ornish's Program for Reversing Heart Disease, by Dr. Dean Ornish

Random House   Price $24.95
201 E. 50th Street
New York, NY 10022

Dr. Ornish discusses using lifestyle changes instead of surgery to reduce the risk of heart disease. The book presents an interesting concept: heart bypass surgery does not affect the *cause* of heart disease, it only bypasses the cause. The condition will return after bypass surgery if patient and doctor do not treat the cause — poor lifestyle habits.

Head First, The Biology of Hope, by Norman Cousins

E. P. Dutton, Inc.   Price $9.95
2 Park Avenue
New York, NY 10016

Cousins describes how he became an active partner with his doctor by thoroughly understanding his condition and treatment plan. He then developed a positive mental attitude to help combat the disease.   Doctor/patient communication and patient attitude can contribute much to the healing process, the author maintains.

Open Heart Surgery, a Guidebook for Patients and Families, by Ina L. Yalof

Random House   Price $11.95
201 E. 50th Street
New York, NY 10022

Yalof discusses the various heart surgery procedures, costs, how surgery is performed and when surgery is indicated.

Managing Your Doctor, by Dr. Arthur S. Freese

Stein and Day Publishers   Price $7.95
Scarborough House   Out of Print
Briarcliff Manor, NY 10510   Available at Library

The title is self-explanatory. The book provides insights on how to deal with your doctor.

Medicine on Trial, by Inlander/Levin/Weiner

Prentice Hall Press   Price $18.95
1230 Avenue of the Americas
New York, NY 10020

This book presents an insider's view of questionable medical practices, errors and arrogance.

The Merck Manual of Diagnosis and Therapy, by Robert Berkoh, M.D.

Merck & Co., Inc.   Price $20.00
P.O. Box 2000
Rahway, NJ 07065

One of the original manuals for professional reference to symptoms, conditions, diagnosis, and suggested therapy.

No More Hysterectomies, by Vicki Hufnagel, M.D.

New American Library   Price $18.95
1633 Broadway
New York, NY 10019

Written by a female surgeon, this book discusses the frequency of hysterectomy surgery and many surgical and non surgical alternatives.

The Patient's Advocate — The Complete Handbook of Patient's Rights, by
   Barbara Huttmann, R.N.

Viking Press   Price $16.95
625 Madison Avenue   Out of Print
New York, NY 10022   Available at Library

   The book, written by a hospital nurse, is based on her experiences in the
hospital. It provides excellent insights into the workings of a hospital from the
viewpoint of a medical insider. It offers suggestions for patients on how to deal
with hospital staff. It also discusses how to guard against mistaken diagnosis,
redundant tests, excessive costs and unnecessary surgery. Sample forms are
provided and your legal rights are discussed. Although this book was published
in 1981, the information is still appropriate for hospital admission ten years later,
since not much has changed.

Physician's Desk Reference, by Edward Barnhart

Medical Economics Company   Price $38.95
680 Kinderkamack Road
Oradell, NJ 07649

   This is the professionals complete guide to prescription drugs providing
warnings, side effects and benefits.

Playing God: The New World of Medical Choices, by Scully, Thomas, and Scully.

Simon and Schuster, Inc.   Price $19.95
Simon and Schuster Building
1230 Avenue of the Americas
New York, NY 10020

   The book discusses health care consumerism. The authors maintain the
consumer has to be more involved in decisions concerning treatment.

The Silent World of Doctor and Patient, by Jay Katz

Free Press/McMillan   Price $9.95
866 Third Avenue
New York, NY 10022

   The book discusses the doctor-patient relationship and encourages more open
dialogue. It suggests that the patient should be more involved with the decision
about his treatment plan and how to get involved.

So Your Doctor Recommended Surgery, by Dr. John Lewis

Dember Books   Price $22.95
80 Eighth Avenue
New York, NY 10011

Many of the most frequently performed surgeries discussed and include indications, alternatives and outcomes. The doctor suggests some surgical procedures to avoid and why.

Take This Book to the Hospital With You: A Consumer's Guide to Surviving Your Hospital Stay, by Charles Inlander

Rodale Press   Price $9.95
33 E. Minor Street
Emmanus, PA 18049

A consumer rights oriented book discussing what you should expect when you visit a hospital and how to protect your rights.

Taking Part: The Survivor's Guide to the Hospital Room, by Donald M. Vicker

The Center for Corporate Health Promotion   Price $19.95
1850 Centennial Park Drive
Reston, VA 22051

The book discusses how the patient can avoid risk in the hospital and outlines when hospitalization is needed. It also discusses patients' rights and responsibility and provides a list of surgeries which can be performed on an outpatient basis. It uses flow charts to assist patients in the decision-making process.

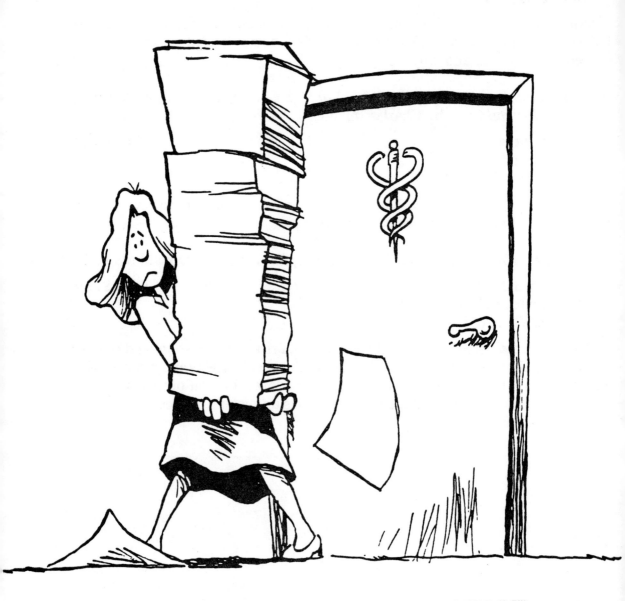

CHAPTER 3

PREPARING FOR DOCTOR VISIT

Most of the questions in this book are designed to address quality issues with your medical provider. You do have a responsibility, however, to provide the physician with complete information so they can make the correct diagnosis and treatment plan. Without the correct information from the patient, even the most qualified provider can't provide the correct treatment.

This section provides a reminder of information the physician will need before determining a course of treatment for you. It is extremely important that you provide your physician with clear and concise information to ensure a correct diagnosis and treatment plan.

Understand, that if you provide *only general information* about your condition or illness, it may be very difficult for the physician to make a diagnosis. This can lead to a *general diagnosis* and a *general treatment plan*. If you provide the physician *very specific* information, then *specific diagnosis* and *specific treatment plan* can be provided.

It is also important that you not be bashful about your condition. Be direct and specific. Include the fact that you may be seeing other doctors and receiving other treatment and medications.

Without specific data, it is very difficult for the physician to make the proper diagnosis. The diagnosis process is closer to an art than a science. After the physician has made an artful decision about your condition, it is then researched, confirmed and treated by the use of science.

Please be prepared to answer the following questions for your physician so that he can fully diagnose your condition or illness and develop a treatment plan.

INFORMATION COMMON TO MOST CONDITIONS AND ILLNESSES

* How many days have you had the problem?

* Have you had this problem before?
  - When?
  - What was the treatment/effect?

* When does the condition occur?
  - Time of day?
  - Activity?
  - How long does it last?
  - Frequency?

* Do you know of anyone else with the same condition?

CONDITIONS

* Pain
  - Where is the pain located?
  - What is the type of pain?
    - Dull, tingling, throbbing?
  - Is the pain constant?
    - To the touch? Only at certain times?

* Skin
  - Where on the skin?
  - Is the skin hot, cold, clammy?
  - Rash, spots?
  - Is it spreading? How fast?

* Fever
  - What is your actual temperature?
  - Does it vary by time of day, activity?
  - Does it alternate with chills?

* Headache
  - Where is the headache located?
    - Behind the eye, one side of head only, top of head, back of neck, forehead?
  - Does it occur only when you stand up?
  - Only after an activity?

- What is the activity?
- Are you taking any new drugs, vitamins or over-the-counter medications?

* Any Discharge?
- Clear, white, yellow, itchy, burning, bloody?

DRUGS

It is extremely important that you thoroughly discuss the medications that you are taking with your physician. If you do not tell the physician what medications you are taking, it is quite possible that he may start to treat the side effects of the medication rather than the actual cause of your condition. This is especially true if you are taking more than three medications at one time. Since all medications have a side effect, the more medications you take, the more side effects you will experience. The more medications you take, the more difficult it is for your physician to determine if your condition results from an illness or drug side effects.

It is also important that you do not take drugs prescribed to other people or drugs which are out-of-date. Prescriptions are very specific to the individual and are based on age, body weight and extent of illness. Body weight, age and race can affect the absorption of the drug. A child will absorb a drug much faster than a senior adult because of different rates of metabolism.

Lastly, you should discuss lifestyle changes that would allow you to reduce your medication. Lifestyle changes have many positive benefits that drugs do not offer.

* What drugs, over-the-counter medications and vitamins are you currently taking? (It is best to bring the bottles with you.)

* What conditions are the drugs treating?

* What is the dosage?

* What is the frequency?

* How long have you been taking the drug?

* Are you allergic to any drugs? Please be specific. Do not confuse the doctor with the difference between a drug allergy and a drug side effect.

  (If you indicate that you have a drug allergy, the physician probably will not consider it as a course of treatment. If you have a drug side effect, you may want to discuss the side effect versus the treatment benefits.)

MEDICAL HISTORY

It is strongly recommended that you take your past medical records with you when you visit your doctor. They contain your medical history and provide a baseline to measure the extent of change caused by your current condition.

With the increased mobility of American society, it is important that you ask your physician for copies of your medical records to give to your new physician at your new location. A polite request to most physicians explaining your need for a complete medical history file should result in your receiving a copy of your medical records, even in states which prohibit patient access to their personal medical records.

* Have you been hospitalized or had previous surgery?
  - Why?
  - When?

* What is your past exposure to x-rays?

* Have you had any blood transfusions?
  - What is your blood type?
  - What is your Rh factor?

* Have you had any exposure to toxic or chemical products?
  - Was it on the job or where you live?

* Prepare a family history. Indicate the medical history of all family members, including diseases, illnesses, deaths.

* Are you currently in an exercise program?
  - Type?
  - Frequency?

* Have you had any recent lifestyle changes?
  - New living quarters?
  - New job/responsibility?
  - Divorce/separation?
  - Problems with children?
  - Personal relationships?
  - Stress?
  - Money/bills?

* Any other recent changes?
  - Diet programs?
  - Weight loss?
  - New animals?
  - New house plants?
  - Change in cleaning supplies?
  - Change in lotions?

-    Change in make-up?
-    Change in medications, vitamins and over-the-counter drugs?

Please provide your physician with as much of this information as possible. This is your chance to give the information needed to properly treat you.

INFORMATION YOUR DOCTOR WILL NEED

1. <u>INFORMATION COMMON TO MOST CONDITIONS AND ILLNESSES</u>
   * How many days have you had the problem?
   * Have you had this problem before?
     - When?
     - What was the treatment/effect?
   * When does the condition occur?
     - Time of day?
     - Activity?
     - How long does it last?
     - Frequency?
   * Do you know of anyone else with the same condition?

2. <u>CONDITIONS</u>
   * Pain
     - Where is the pain located?
     - What is the type of pain?
       - Dull, tingling, throbbing?
     - Is the pain constant?
       - To the touch, only at certain times?
   * Skin
     - Where on the skin?
     - Is the skin hot, cold, clammy?
     - Rash, spots?
     - Is it spreading? How fast?
   * Fever
     - What is your actual temperature?
     - Does it vary by time of day, activity?
     - Does it alternate with chills?
   * Headache
     - Where is the headache located?
       - Behind the eye, one side of head only, top of head, back of neck, forehead?
     - Does it occur only when you stand up?
     - Only after an activity?
     - What is the activity?
     - Are you taking any new drugs, vitamins, or over-the-counter medications?
   * Any Discharge
     - Clear, white, yellow, itchy, burning, bloody?

3. <u>DRUGS</u>
   * What drugs, over-the-counter medications and vitamins are you currently taking? (It is best to bring the bottles with you.)

3. <u>DRUGS</u> - Continued
   * What conditions are the drugs treating?
   * What is the dosage?
   * What is the frequency?
   * How long have you been taking the drug?
   * Are you allergic to any drugs? Please be specific. Do not confuse the doctor with the difference between a drug allergy and a drug side effect.

4. <u>HISTORY</u>
   * Have you been hospitalized or had previous surgery?
     - Why?
     - When?
   * What is your past exposure to x-rays?
   * Have you had any blood transfusions?
     - What is your blood type?
     - What is your Rh factor?
   * Have you had any exposure to toxic or chemical products?
     - Was it on the job or where you live?
   * Prepare a family history. Indicate the medical history of all family members, including diseases, illnesses, deaths.
   * Currently in an exercise program?
     - Type?
     - Frequency?
   * Any recent lifestyle changes?
     - New living quarters?
     - New job/responsibility?
     - Divorce/separation?
     - Problems with children?
     - Personal relationships?
     - Stress?
     - Money/bills?
   * Any other recent changes?
     - Diet programs?
     - Weight loss?
     - New animals?
     - New house plants?
     - Change in cleaning supplies?
     - Change in lotions?
     - Change in make-up?
     - Change in medications, vitamins and over-the-counter drugs?

Reorder from: MED. ED. Inc., P.O. Box 40696, Mesa, Arizona 85274-0496, (602) 345-1943

NOTES

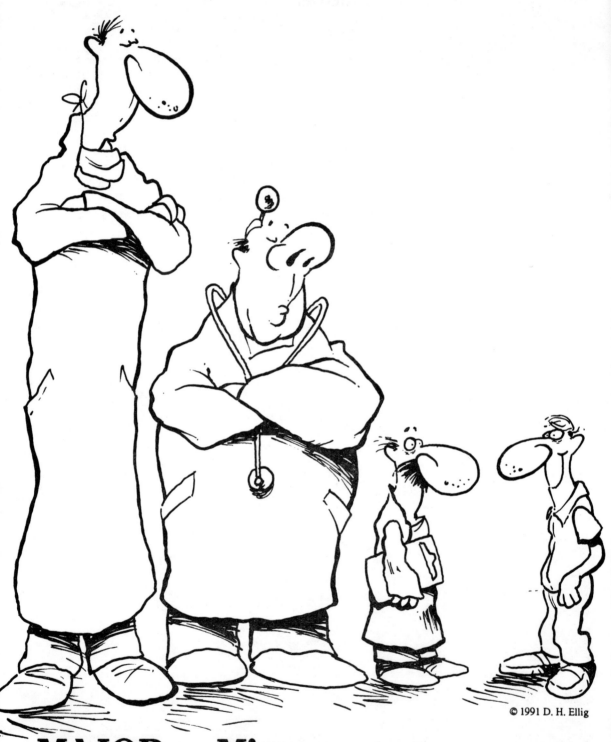

© 1991 D. H. Ellig

MAJOR DEITY   **Minor Deity**   Doctor   Patient

CHAPTER 4

PATIENT PATIENT

Patient is a word that can be used as an adjective to modify itself as a noun. Which is your definition of a patient?

Patient as:

An Adjective

1. Bearing or enduring pain, trouble, especially without complaining or losing self-control.
2. Refusing to be provoked or angered by an insult; forebearing; tolerant.
3. Calmly tolerating delay, confusion, inefficiency, etc.
4. Able to wait calmly for something desired.
5. Showing or characterized by patience.
6. Steady; diligent; persevering.

A Noun

1. A person receiving care or treatment, esp. from a doctor

Many patients unfortunately feel they are patient (adj.) patients. What patients (n.) need are patient (adj. 2, 3, 4, or 6) doctors, not M.D.'s (Minor Deities). Occasionally you will meet a MAJOR DEITY (a Minor Deity suffering from testosterone poisoning). A major deity finds it very difficult to treat mere mortals as equal partners as they know everything and are always right.

*Definitions courtesy Webster's Dictionary, 3rd College Edition, 1988.

An Informed Patient...

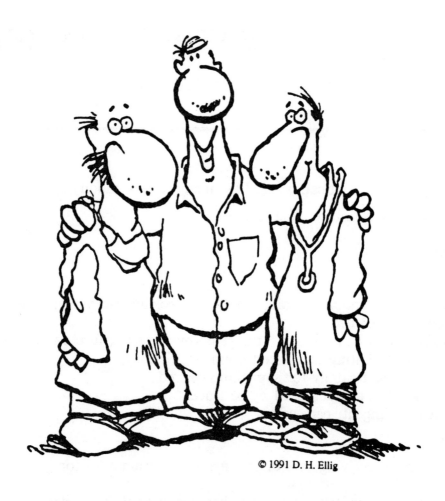

© 1991 D. H. Ellig

Is An Equal Partner.

CHAPTER 5

WHAT YOU SHOULD
REALLY BE TOLD

Many patients don't know they have the right to be fully informed. These rights are protected by the Informed Consent Doctrine and the AMA Code of Ethics. This chapter will discuss these rights so that as a patient you will not be intimidated, you will know that the care giver has a legal, ethical, and moral obligation to answer your questions. You need only to have the courage to ask.

Many patients sign consent forms without reading them, never fully understanding the nature of the surgical procedure nor the rights and liabilities involved with it. The purpose of this chapter is to take a closer look at medical consent forms to help patients become active informed participants in the healthcare decision-making process. While this chapter discusses consent forms in detail, informed consent is really a process of dialogue between patient and doctor, not just a form. The form should merely serve as a written reminder of the discussion topics and data provided by the doctor to the patient.

THE INFORMED CONSENT DOCTRINE

"The root premise is the concept, fundamental in American Jurisprudence, that '[e]very human being of adult years and sound mind has a right to determine what shall be done with his own body . . . .' True consent to what happens to one's self is the *informed exercise of a choice,* and that entails an *opportunity to evaluate knowledgeably* the *options available* and the *risks* attendant upon each."
— *Canterbury v. Spence*

The definition of informed consent is changing from one of "standard of care" to "right of self-determination." "Standard of care" is defined as the community standard established by the physicians in the local community. This means that the "standard of care" could and did vary from community to community. "Standard of care" was what the physician thought it should be, not what the patient understood.

The "right to self-determination" doctrine of informed consent changes informed consent from physician-based understanding to patient-based understanding. Informed consent now means that the patient can provide informed consent only if the patient fully understands the procedure, risk, and complications. The explanation of procedures, risks and complications should not be so ambiguous that the patient cannot understand his/her choices.

Therefore, the doctor and the patient share the responsibility to *understand.* The doctor must communicate in simple words and the patient *must* tell the doctor they *don't understand* or the doctor will assume the patient does understand the diagnosis and treatment plan.

What Should Be Explained?

Before the patient can give informed consent, the following information should be provided for *all* diagnostic tests, and medical and surgical procedures:

1. Expected outcome of diagnostic test.
2. Diagnosis of the patient.
3. Nature, purpose and benefits of treatment/test.
4. Risk/consequences of treatment/test.
    (Remote consequences of risk for the normal patient do not normally require discussion. If, however, the risk result is severe, such as death or disability, it should be discussed. If normal risks become high because of patient history, it should be discussed. Consequences should include both temporary and permanent affects upon the patient, such as discomfort, disability, and/or disfigurement.)
5. Probability of success.
    (Patient should also determine what are the parameters of success.)
6. The permanent results of the treatment/test.
    (These should include such items as scars and discussion of future care.)
7. Alternative treatments.
8. Prognosis if not treated.

The Problems

Even though the informed consent doctrine is changing from physician-based to patient-based, and case law has provided detailed patient information parameters, the standard informed consent form has not been changed to provide the patient with the information needed to make an informed decision.

The content of most informed consent forms are so ambiguous, lacking in detail, and difficult to understand that the patient cannot give informed consent.

Ambiguous

Most consent forms are ambiguous. The patient gives consent for a specific procedure which is later expanded by words such as "necessary and advisable or unforeseen." These words are normally explained as being necessary to give the physician an opportunity to perform additional procedures in the event of a "medical emergency." The problem with this explanation is that the informed consent doctrine allows the physician to give emergency care without patient consent. The words "necessary and advisable or unforeseen" allow the physician to perform additional procedures that he deems "necessary and advisable or unforeseen," but which may not be a true medical emergency, but rather a matter of convenience. The words also allow the physician to defend the additional surgery by stating that the patient gave informed consent and the procedures were deemed "necessary and advisable" by the physician.

Lacking in Detail

Most consent forms have a clause that states the nature, purpose, consequences, risk, complications and alternative treatments that have been explained and that the patient understands.

The problem is the form does not show **what** was explained, actually told, shown or provided to the patient. There is no documented backup of the doctor/patient discussion which led the patient to sign the consent form, nor is there any attachment or addendum which provides these details.

This, then, leads to difficulty in resolving disputes. It is quite possible the two parties will have different stories of the verbal conversations.

Readability

Not only are most consent forms ambiguous and lacking in detail, but most of the population cannot understand them because the text readability is difficult.

A study of over 1,000 consent forms to perform experimental studies revealed that only 7 percent were written at the readability level found in Time Magazine. The other 93 percent of the forms were written at these readability levels:

    21% — equal to a scientific journal
    56% — equal to an academic magazine
    17% — equal to Atlantic Monthly

What's Being Done

Many physicians now have more detailed discussions with patients about suggested treatment plans. This process will make the doctor and patient equal partners in the decision to treat or not to treat. The expectations of outcomes, in addition, will be clearer to the patient.

A survey indicated that 80 to 90 percent of the physicians always or usually discuss the following points with their patients:

Diagnosis   Alternate treatment modes
Reservations concerning the diagnosis   Risk consequences of alternate treatment
Nature of the treatment   Benefits of alternate treatment
Purpose of treatment   Probability of success
Risk of treatment   Pros and cons of alternate treatment vs.
Negative psychological consequences   recommended treatment
Benefits of treatment   Impact on patient's family
Probability of success   Impact on patient's job
                                            Prognosis if no treatment

Less frequently discussed are the cost of treatment or cost of alternative treatments or what portion insurance will cover.

The time physicians allotted to discuss 21 issues is shown below:

Minutes	% of Doctors	Cumulative %
0 – 5	21	21
6 – 10	25	46
11 – 15	23	69
16 – 20	13	81
more than 20	19	100

Less than 70 percent of physicians spent 15 minutes or less discussing 21 important treatment issues. It should not be surprising then that 33 percent of the physicians indicate that the patients have very little or no recollection of the discussion (a good reason for taking notes or recording the discussions), 57 percent remember only the significant points and only 10 percent of the patients remember most of the discussion.

Benefits to Informed Consent

If a patient is more fully informed, both the patient and the physician need to spend more time in discussion. There are significant benefits to both the physician and the patient if the patient is fully informed. The first is that the patient who fully understands his treatment plan can fully cooperate with the physician and carry out his treatment responsibilities. Studies have shown that the best patient is the patient who is psychologically involved. A fully informed patient will be less likely to have doctor/patient conflicts concerning treatment outcomes.

Review of Forms

This chapter will review four forms, two of which protect the doctor and hospital, and two of which protect the patient.

Surgical Consent Form — Protects Physician
Hospital Admittance Form — Protects Hospital
Informed Consent Checklist Form (New) — Protects Patient
The Patient's Bill of Rights — Gives Patients Rights While in the Hospital

The *Surgical Consent Form* is an authorization to perform surgical procedures on the patient. Its purpose is to protect the physician by having the patient acknowledge that the doctor has informed the patient of risks, complications and consequences of the doctor's treatment.

The *Hospital Admittance Form* covers the hospital's responsibility, nursing care, theft, teaching programs, release of information, medical power of attorney, releases the hospital from the doctor's actions, and includes the patient's responsibility to pay for services rendered. This form does more to protect the hospital than it does to protect the patient.

Both the Surgical Consent Form and the Hospital Admittance Forms basically say "I told you, you can't blame me, you had full knowledge." Many times the doctor and patient discuss the issues addressed on consent forms in generalities. The *Informed Consent Checklist Form* is more specific and creates fewer misunderstandings.

The *Informed Consent Checklist Form* serves as an in-depth written inventory of important information and issues agreed to on the consent forms and as a reminder of important patient issues. The form was designed to provide a source for the patient to record all the issues that are referenced on the doctor/hospital forms, but which in the past where never recorded by the patient, but may have been covered verbally only in very general, nonspecific terms by the doctor and hospital. If the form is completed, the patient will be truly "informed," so that consent may be given. It can be the patient's counterpart to the physician and hospital forms.

The *Informed Consent Checklist Form* is important for those individuals who must make a decision for their children, loved ones, or adult parents. It specifically documents information referenced and/or consented to on the *Surgical Consent Form* and *Hospital Admittance Form*.

The *Patient's Bill of Rights* was developed by the American Hospital Association. It encompasses a broad range of patient rights and issues. Its purpose is to promote more effective care and greater satisfaction for the patient, the physician and the hospital organization.

THE SURGICAL CONSENT FORM

The *Surgical Consent Form* serves as the patient's legal authorization for the physician and/or his associates to perform surgical procedures. Its function is to release the doctor from the effects of miscommunication between doctor and patient.

The form states that the patient has been *fully informed* of the purpose and nature of the surgical procedure, *understands the risks* and/or complications involved, is aware of possible alternative methods of treatment, and *willingly accepts* the consequences.

You should read and thoroughly understand the consequences of signing the form before signing it. It is a legal contract. Your signing it indicates you understand the consequences. If the form contains any language or issues you do not understand, you should ASK QUESTIONS and REQUEST ASSISTANCE from your health care providers. You and your doctor will be glad you did.

The following overview of the *Surgical Consent Form* is designed to acquaint you with consent form issues and discuss the consequences of "uninformed consent." Remember, you have the right to question and the power to amend those areas that are not clear or which you do not accept. (The sample consent form shown contains the most common language found in consent forms. **It does not meet the requirement of Informed Consent Doctrine** without more written documentation showing **what** was discussed.)

The *Surgical Consent Form* is not an irrevocable document, you may revoke consent at any time. If you change your mind, you can change the form.

The two greatest areas of concern on the *Surgical Consent Form* are items 1 and 2. When we agree to surgery we assume that *our doctor will do the surgery* we discussed. The consent form says *any doctor can do any surgery.* You can simply change items 1 and 2 by saying "But doctor, didn't we agree you would do the surgery we discussed, if I sign the consent form provided it says any doctor can do any surgery. I don't want that, I want to be informed."

No. 1   This authorizes your doctor to perform the surgical procedure. It also allows him/her to delegate the procedure to an associate or assistant. This statement allows your physician great latitude to elect to delegate your procedure to someone else, assist rather than conduct, teach others under his guidance, or to not even be present at your surgery. If you wish to grant surgery authorization to your doctor only, state so on the form. If you are comfortable with your doctor and his qualifications, you may want to insist that only your doctor perform the surgery.

Note: AMA Ethics state, "to have another physician operate on one's patient without the patient's knowledge and consent is a deceit."

No. 2   This indicates that the physician and his associates may perform additional procedures that may not have been discussed with you, that you may not have approved and whose consequences you may not want. You can limit additional surgical procedures to *medical emergency only* rather than physician elective procedures. The words "unforseen" give the physician more latitude and are not the same as medical emergency.

No. 3   This statement gives total control of your anesthesia to the anesthesiologist. If you have discussed the method of administration and type of anesthetic, you should so note here. Changes may be made in the event of a medical emergency.

No. 4   This item indicates that you have been fully informed and are fully aware of the risk of the administration of anesthesia. Have you been informed and do you have written documentation? Most patients don't meet their anesthesiologist until they are in the operating room, at which time it is too late to be "fully informed."

No. 5   This confirms that you are aware of any possible consequences, risks involved, or alternative methods of treatment and do not require any further explanation. To become this fully informed, you will need to do some extensive research. Thoroughly consider and research your alternatives before signing such an important authorization.

No. 6   Consent to this only after you have received the pathologist's report indicating surgery was necessary. This item allows the hospital authorities to use your tissues and cells in any way they feel is appropriate. This may include research or for-profit sales. You can address this issue if you so desire.

No. 7   This states that your primary care physician has no responsibility for the actions of those physicians whom he selected to be members of your surgical team, and places the primary responsibility on you for their actions. Have you investigated the quality and training of the other team members or have you requested your primary care physician to accept the responsibility for the team members he selected?

No. 8   This statement acknowledges that you have the right to amend the contract and have done so before signing. To verify all amended issues, initial all changes and/or amendments.

No. 9   The final item verifies that your physician has fully informed you of all aspects of the procedure. Keep in mind that this could include verbal conversations as well as written documentation. If a patient/doctor dispute arises in the future and the patient has received no written documentation, the doctor notes recorded in the doctor's file will be the basis for settlement. The patient might want to record verbal conversations on the *Informed Consent Checklist Form* discussed later in this chapter.

SAMPLE SURGICAL CONSENT FORM

PIENT: _____ DATE: _____ TIME: _____ a.m. / p.m.

I authorize the performance of the following operation(s) or procedure(s) _____

_____

_____

(state nature and extent of each operation or other procedure)

to be performed by Dr._____ and **associates and assistants of his choice[1]** on the above-named patient.

I consent to the performance of operations and procedures **in addition to or different from those now contemplated,[2]** whether or not arising from presently unforseen conditions, which the above-named doctor and his associates or assistants may consider necessary or advisable in the course of the operation.

I consent to the **administration of such anesthetics as may be considered necessary[3]** or advisable with the exception of _____

(if none, **write** none)

I understand that the **administration of anesthesia involves some risk to the patient[4]**, even though done in a careful and prudent manner. I understand that an outpatient should not engage in activities requiring judgement and/or fine coordination or take any depressant drugs like alcohol or tranquilizers for at least twenty-four (24) hours following an anesthetic. Residual effects may last for several days.

I confirm the following: that my physicians have explained to me the nature, purpose and **possible consequences of each operation** or procedure **as well as risks involved, possible complications and possible alternative methods of treatment**; that I understand that the explanation I have received is not exhaustive and that other, more remote risks and consequences may arise; that I have been advised that a more detailed and complete explanation of any of the foregoing matters will be given me if I so desire; **that I do not desire such further explanation;[5]** and that I acknowledge that I have reached no guarantees or assurances from anyone as to the results that may be obtained.

I consent to the **disposal by hospital authorities of any tissues[6]** which may have been removed.

I understand that the above-named physician and his associates or assistants will be occupied solely with performing such operation or procedure and **the physicians in attendance at such operation** or procedure for the purpose of **administering anesthesia**, and the physician or physicians performing services involving **pathology and radiology**, may not be the agents, servants or employees of the above-named hospital nor of any surgeon, but may be independent contractors.**[7]**

I understand that natural teeth, restorations, and prosthetics are all subject to accidental damage, even with careful anesthetic and surgical management. Also I have been advised that all removable teeth should be removed before going to surgery; then I agree the responsibility for loss or damage will be mine if I fail to remove such teeth.

I acknowledge that all blank spaces to this document have been either completed or **crossed off prior to my signing.[8]**

(CROSS OUT AND INITIAL ANY PARAGRAPHS ABOVE, WHICH DO NOT APPLY)

_____
(Patient)

_____
(Witness)

If patient is unable to consent by reason of age or some other factor, state reasons: _____

_____

_____

_____	_____
Witness	Signature of legally authorized rep.
_____	_____
Witness	Relationship to patient

PHYSICIAN'S STATEMENT

I certify that I have informed the above-named patient to the following: The nature, **purpose and possible consequences of the operation or procedure, risks involved, possibilities of complications, and possible alternative methods of treatment.[9]**

DATE: _____   _____
                                        Physician

THE HOSPITAL CONSENT FORM

The *Hospital Consent Form* serves two purposes: to assure that the patient agrees to relieve the hospital from actions of others not employed by the hospital (the doctors providing services) and to act as the financial agreement between the patient and hospital.

The form verifies that the patient is primarily responsible for payment and that financial arrangements will be made prior to discharge.

It is suggested that you carefully review and understand the issues raised in this document.

No. 1   This permits the hospital to provide services directed by your physician. If you and your doctor are to be a team, you may want to indicate that the doctor orders may be reviewed by you and that you have the right to refuse any treatment you desire.

No. 2   This releases the hospital from accepting responsibility for actions of the physicians or nonhospital employees. The hospital would like to remove itself from the actions of healthcare providers to whom they have granted admitting or staff privileges. Did you select and qualify these providers or did the hospital? If the hospital selected these providers of services, cross out this statement so hospital maintains responsibility or ask the hospital to provide qualification data so you can make an informed provider decision. Notice that both the *Surgical Consent Form* and the *Hospital Admittance Form* protect each of them from action by others. How does the patient protect himself? See the *Informed Consent Checklist Form*.

No. 3   This item indicates that you may receive treatment provided by individuals in training (interns and residents). If you prefer treatment be provided only by qualified practitioners and individuals whom you have previously met, cross out this statement. This may be especially pertinent in June or july when medical schools graduate new doctors.

No. 4   This item gives the doctor and hospital permission to take photographs and videotape of your surgical procedure. If a videotape is to be made, can you have a copy for your records?

No. 5   Many times patients have difficulty getting access to their medical records. This statement indicates that the patient has the right to access those medical records. If you want a copy of your medical records or want to look at your medical records, you may do so. In some states, patients do not have access to their own records. Notice how many people and organizations are allowed to access patient medical records, including the patient, with this *Hospital Admittance Form*.

If you wish, you may make this release valid for only one or two years.

No. 6   This grants the release of your medical information for medical studies and research. If you disagree or profit is involved, you may want to discuss the possibility of patient participation.

No. 7   A recent federal law requires that hospitals provide patients with information concerning Living Wills or medical power of attorneys. Please refer to the chapter on Living Wills for a more complete discussion.

No. 8   This statement says that the patient need only make arrangements to pay the hospital bill. The patient is *not required to pay* the hospital bill prior to discharge.

No. 9   This item entitles the hospital to collect insurance payments for application toward the patient's bill. It is possible that the hospital could collect twice if a patient has an individual medical policy and an employer group policy. Traditionally, the individual and group policies do not coordinate benefits. Coordination of benefits means that only 100 percent of the bill will be paid not 200 percent.

atient or someone acting for the patient agrees to the following terms of hospital admission:

MEDICAL TREATMENT: Patient will be treated by his/her attending doctor or specialists. Patient **authorizes Hospital to perform services ordered by the doctors.**[1] Special consent forms may be needed. **Many doctors and assistants** (such as those providing x-rays, lab tests, and anesthesiology) may not be Hospital employees and **are responsible for their own treatment activities.**[2] Patient consents to the treatment to be provided by those doctors and technicians.

GENERAL DUTY NURSING: Hospital provides only general nursing care. If the patient needs special or private nursing, it must be arranged by the patient or by the doctor treating the patient.

MONEY AND VALUABLES: The Hospital has a safe in which to keep money or valuables. It will not be responsible for any loss or damage to items not deposited in the safe. The Hospital will not be responsible for loss or damage to items such as glasses, dentures, hearing aids and contact lenses.

TEACHING PROGRAMS: The Hospital participates in programs for training of healthcare personnel. Some services may be provided to the patient by **persons in training** under the supervision and instruction of doctors or hospital employees.[3] These persons may also observe care given to the patient by doctors and hospital employees. **Photos or video tapes may be made of surgical procedures.**[4]

RELEASE OF INFORMATION: The Hospital **may disclose all or any part of the patient's medical and/or financial records** (INCLUDING INFORMATION REGARDING ALCOHOL OR DRUG ABUSE) to the following:

a. **Third Parties:** Including, but not limited to any person or corporation, or their designee, which may be liable under a contract to the hospital, the patient, a family member, or employer of the patient, for payment of all or part of the hospital's charges, such as insurance companies, workers' compensation payers, hospital or medical service companies, welfare funds, governmental agencies or the patient's employer; quality assurance and peer review committees, subcommittees ad hocs or consultants; utilization review organizations, medicare review organizations; medicare review organizations, hospital accrediting surveyors; treating physicians; and hospital and treating physician's professional liability insurance carriers.[5]

b. **Medical Audit:** The Hospital conducts a program of medical audit and the patient's medical information may be reviewed and released by employees, members of the medical staff or other authorized persons to appropriate agencies as part of this program.

c. **Medical Research:** Information may be **released for use in medical studies and medical research.**[6]

d. **Other Healthcare Providers:** Information may be released to other healthcare providers for continued patient care.

I understand that the authorization granted in items 5. a, b, c and d may be revoked by me at any time, except to the extent to which action has been taken in reliance upon it. The authorization will stay in effect as long as the need for information in items 5. a, b, c and d exist.

ave read and understand this Admissions Agreement, have received a copy and I am the patient, the parent of a minor child or the court appointed ardian for the patient and am authorized to act on the patient's behalf to sign this Agreement.

_____ _____
WITNESS PATIENT PARENT OF MINOR CHILD COURT APPOINTED GUARDIAN
(PLEASE CIRCLE THE CORRECT TITLE)

_____
DATE TIME

MEDICAL POWER OF ATTORNEY: I appoint _____

_____ _____
ADDRESS PHONE

s my agent to act in all matters relating to my health care, including full power to give or refuse consent to all medical, surgical nd hospital care. This power of attorney shall be effective upon my disability or incapacity or when there is uncertainty, whether am dead or alive, and shall have the same effect as if I were alive, competent, and able to act for myself.[7]

_____ _____
WITNESS **FINANCIAL AGREEMENT** PATIENT

agree that in return for the services provided to the patient, I will **pay the account of the patient,** and/or prior to discharge **make financial rrangements**[8] satisfactory to the hospital for payment. If the account is sent to an attorney for collection, I agree to pay reasonable attorney's fees nd collection expenses. The amount of the attorney's fee shall be established by the Court and not by a Jury in any court action. A delinquent account ay be charged interest at the legal rate.

request that payment of any authorized Medicare benefits be made on my behalf. I assign the benefits payable for physician services to the physician r organization furnishing the services or authorize such physician or organization to submit a claim to Medicare for payment to me.

any signer is entitled to benefits of any type whatsoever under any policy insuring patient, or any other party liable to patient, e benefits are hereby assigned to hospital or to the provider group rendering service, for application on patient's bill. However, **T IS UNDERSTOOD THAT THE UNDERSIGNED AND PATIENT ARE PRIMARILY RESPONSIBLE FOR PAYMENT F PATIENT'S BILL.**[9]

GRANTING ADMISSION OR RENDERING TREATMENT, THE HOSPITAL IS RELYING ON MY AGREEMENT TO PAY THE ACCOUNT. MERGENCY CARE WILL BE PROVIDED WITHOUT REGARD TO THE ABILITY TO PAY.

_____ _____
PATIENT OTHER PARTY AGREEING TO PAY

_____ _____
WITNESS RELATIONSHIP TO PATIENT

_____
DATE

RISK ASSESSMENT

The *Informed Consent Checklist Form* on the next page serves as a reminder of the medical treatment information to be provided by medical case law and AMA Ethics Standards before a patient may give legal consent. The form addresses the legal, ethical and moral obligations of the healthcare provider. It is the physician's legal and ethical obligation to make sure the patient understands the procedures, risk and complications. The physician also has an ethical and moral obligation to reveal the financial and personal relationships with any of the healthcare providers. (AMA Ethics state, "The physician has an affirmative ethical obligation to disclose his ownership of a health facility to his patient . . . .) It is the patient counterpart to the *Surgical Consent Form*. This form provides a written record of what the patient and the physician consent to when they sign the *Surgical Consent Form*, i.e., the typical physician's *Surgical Consent Form* has a statement to the effect "My physician has explained to me the nature, purpose, possible consequences and complications of each procedure, and possible alternative treatment methods as well as the risk involved."

The physician also certifies that, "I have informed the patient of the nature, purpose and possible consequences of the operation or procedure, risk involved, possibilities of complications and possible alternate methods of treatment." The *Informed Consent Checklist Form* documents the facts behind the patient and doctor statements.

The *Informed Consent Checklist Form* is very simple and logical. It records the information verbally provided by the physician to the patient:

It lists the alternate treatment plans discussed.
It quantifies the risk and complications of the procedure selected.
It lists other information, so that the patient may truly provide "informed" consent.

WARNING — It is suggested that you inform the physician that you want to use the *Informed Consent Checklist* before the physician commits to a decision or makes a recommendation.

No professional likes to have his judgment questioned. If you address the issues on the form before a professional judgment is given, the patient and the physician can make a joint informed decision without the patient appearing to challenge the physician's judgment.

The *Informed Consent Checklist,* should be presented with a great deal of tact and an expression of concern for your welfare. Do not use the form to offend the physician.

Use Tact, Don't Attack!

The form may be presented in a **quietly assertive manner**, just as in the past the patient was quietly passive. If the patient needs some support for the use of the *Informed Consent Checklist*, they can simply say, "my insurance company or employer require it." This may, or may not be true.

The patient and the physician should be happy to discuss the issues on the *Informed Consent Checklist*, since it shows both parties agree to a full understanding of the proposed treatment, the risk, complications and outcomes. Such information is required by law if the patient is to give "informed consent."

The open dialogue required to complete the *Informed Consent Checklist Form* should result in less misunderstanding between doctor/patient. The patient's outcome expectations should equal the doctor's, which could reduce a major cause of medical malpractice claims.

Any reservations about signing the form by either party should be thoroughly discussed. The lack of a signature could indicate that the physician and patient do not fully agree about what the surgical consent form says they understand. Some doctors may not agree to sign the form because it is *too* specific and they have not had to in the past, or feel uncomfortable about releasing all the information.

If the physician will not sign the *Informed Consent Checklist Form*, the patient should record as much data as possible to document what was discussed. **There is simply too much important data provided in the risk form to ignore this procedure.**

A Note For Doctors Only

The form on the next page may be the best malpractice policy you don't have to buy!

You no longer will have to defend yourself with "I did too tell you," and the patient responding "You did not, prove it." You will have proof that the patient was fully informed of the risks, possible complications and expected outcomes.

You may even want to try to negotiate a discount on your rate if you use this form as nuisance claims should drop sharply. Claims filed against you should be only for the "true" negligent acts, which are rare.

RISK ASSESSMENT

An Informed Consent Checklist

(Issues to be discussed with physician/hospital administrator in charge of treatment)

Name/Description

Doctor _____ Diagnosis Code _____ _____

Patient _____ Procedure Code _____ _____

Scheduled Surgery Date _____ Estimated Fee _____

TREATMENT INFORMATION: Risk Assessment for above procedure code: _____

Risks: %_____ Cured   %_____ Not Cured   %_____ Disabled   %_____ Death   %_____ Complications

Complications %_____ Infections   %_____ Excessive Bleeding %_____ 2nd Operation   %_____ Other   Explain (on attachment)

Reoccurrence Possibility:

%_____ Need same treatment again in _____ years %_____ Need Different Treatment   %_____ No Additional Treatment

Alternate Treatment No. 1: Risk Assessment for procedure code: _____   Estimated Fee _____

Risks: %_____ Cured   %_____ Not Cured   %_____ Disabled   %_____ Death   %_____ Complications

Complications %_____ Infections   %_____ Excessive Bleeding %_____ 2nd Operation   %_____ Other   Explain (on attachment)

Reoccurrence Possibility:

%_____ Need same treatment again in _____ years %_____ Need Different Treatment   %_____ No Additional Treatment

Alternate Treatment No. 2: Risk Assessment for procedure code: _____   Estimated Fee _____

Risks: %_____ Cured   %_____ Not Cured   %_____ Disabled   %_____ Death   %_____ Complications

Complications %_____ Infections   %_____ Excessive Bleeding %_____ 2nd Operation   %_____ Other   Explain (on attachment)

Reoccurrence Possibility:

%_____ Need same treatment again in _____ years %_____ Need Different Treatment   %_____ No Additional Treatment

Blood Usage Information:

Transfusion (Circle) — Own, Blood Bank, Friends/Relative Donations

Blood Storage — Store Own Blood _____   Intra Operative — Reuse Patient's Blood _____

Implanted Devices Information:

Manufacturer _____   Model No. _____

Any Manufacturer Warnings/Recalls _____   Any FDA Warnings/Recalls _____

Please provide written details: _____

After Surgery Information:

Medication Name _____

Effects _____

Length of Time Taken _____

Lifestyle Changes to Expect/Side Effects _____

TESTING INFORMATION:

Lab Testing Accuracy _____%   Licensed by state? yes [ ] no [ ] Licensed by Medicare yes [ ] no [ ]

Samples will be tested by: [ ] Technician Trainee [ ] Technician [ ] Technologist [ ] Toxicologist [ ] Physician [ ] Pathologist

Imaging (x-ray, ultra sound, CT scan, MRI) will be interpreted by:

[ ] Technician [ ] Ltd. Technician [ ] Practical Technician [ ] Physician [ ] Board-Certified Physician

DOCTOR INFORMATION:

No. times doctor has performed this procedure _____   No. times assistant surgeon has performed this procedure _____

Can patient expect to resume normal lifestyle activities? yes [ ]   no [ ]

    No — Which one _____   Percent of Change _____%

What body functions may patient lose _____   What % _____

Anesthesia Information:

Type — local, block, general, general with intubation _____   Doctor's Name _____

Name of Agent _____   Manufacturer _____ Lot # _____

Risk _____   Complication _____ % of Occurrence _____

Any Warnings: Manufacturer _____   FDA _____

Optional Doctor Information:

Medical School Graduated From _____

Board Specialty _____   Fellowship Designation _____

I (do not [ ]) (do [ ]) agree to waive fees considered "excessive" or "inappropriate" by the insurance company.

Doctor (does not [ ]) (does [ ]) have a financial interest at referred hospital (*i.e.*, loans, ownership, investment, financial incentives, discount office space).

Doctor (does not [ ]) (does [ ]) have a financial interest in referred labs.

(CROSS OUT AND INITIAL ANY PARAGRAPHS ABOVE OR BELOW WHICH DO NOT APPLY.)

acknowledge that I have discussed the above issues with the patient and that in my professional opinion based on training and experience the recommended ocedure has the best risk/benefits outcome for the patient.

Doctor _____

Witness _____   Date _____

HOSPITAL INFORMATION:

Number of times this procedure performed at (hospital name) _____

% Successful _____%   % With Complications _____%

Hospital Mortality Rate _____   Hospital Complication Rate _____   Hospital Infection Rate _____

JCAHO Hospital Accreditation is: Accredited _____   Conditional _____   Not Accredited _____

Doctors (do not [ ]) (do [ ]) have a financial interest at referred hospital (i.e., loans, ownership, investment, financial incentives, discount office space)

Hospital Equipment/Devices Information:

Please provide the following for any devices, equipment, agents which will be used during patient's treatment:

Any manufacturer warnings/recalls _____   Manufacturer _____   Model/Lot No. _____

Any FDA warnings/recalls _____   Corrected?   yes [ ]   no [ ]

Radiology Department is accredited by American College of Radiology?   yes [ ]   no [ ]

Doctors and staff (do not [ ]) (do [ ]) have training/experience to operate equipment used during treatment.

Hospital (does not [ ]) (does [ ]) have a drug testing program for physicians and operating room staff.

(CROSS OUT AND INITIAL ANY PARAGRAPHS ABOVE OR BELOW WHICH DO NOT APPLY.)

also certify, that to the best of my knowledge, neither myself nor the rest of the surgical team has had their license suspended, revoked, or censured by any er organization (state or county medical society) or governing body (board of medical examiners), or is currently before such peer organization or governing ard.

doctor/hospital administrator cannot so certify, please provide details as an attachment.

ospital Administrator _____   Doctor _____

itness _____   Witness _____

ate _____   Date _____

AMERICAN HOSPITAL ASSOCIATION'S
PATIENT'S BILL OF RIGHTS

The *Informed Consent Checklist Form* asks for written information which traditionally has been requested by only a few patients. The *American Hospital Association's Patient's Bill of Rights* gives the patient the right to most of the information requested by the *Informed Consent Checklist Form.*

If the hospital is accredited by JCAHO (Joint Commission on the Accreditation of Health Care Organizations), it must provide the patient with a copy of the *Patient's Bill of Rights* as shown and adhere to the *Bill of Rights* as a part of their hospital accreditation process.

No. 1   The patient does have a right to expect a reasonable explanation of his diagnosis, treatment and outcome in nonmedical terms. The patient has a right to the outcome data requested on the *Informed Consent Checklist Form.*

No. 2   The patient has the right to full information of medically significant risk in terms he can understand. Many patients do not receive written documentation of the possible risk or complications of the suggested treatment. The patient has the right to request this and should.

No. 3   The patient also has the right to receive documentation concerning the alternative treatment programs. It is suggested that the patient also receive a list of the pros and cons of the alternate treatment plans, in order to make an informed decision and give informed consent.

No. 4   The patient may refuse any medical treatment he does not wish, even if it violates the doctor's orders.

No. 5   The patient also has the right to choose who will provide treatment and can decline treatment by those in training at the hospital. Healthcare providers must have the patient's permission.

No. 6   The patient has the right to information about professional (financial) relationships between the doctors and the hospital or the hospital and any research programs.

No. 7   The patient has the right to be aware of experimental treatment and to give his informed consent if these treatments are offered to him.

No. 8   The patient has the right to request a detailed bill rather than simply a summary level bill.

NOTE: Medicare patients have another federally mandated Bill of Rights

The American Hospital Association presents a Patient's Bill of Rights with the expectation that observance of these rights will contribute to more effective patient care and greater satisfaction for the patient, his physician and the hospital organization. Further, the Association presents these rights in the expectation that they will be supported by the hospital on behalf of its patients as an integral part of the healing process. It is recognized that a personal relationship between the physician and the patient is essential for the provision of proper medical care. The traditional physician/patient relationship takes on a new dimension when care is rendered within an organizational structure. Legal precedent has established that the institution itself also has a responsibility to the patient. It is in recognition of these factors that these rights are affirmed.

1.   The patient has the right to considerate and respectful care.

2.   The patient has the **right to obtain from his physician complete current information concerning his diagnosis, treatment and prognosis in terms the patient can be reasonably expected to understand.**[1] When it is not medically advisable to give such information to the patient, the information should be made available to an appropriate person in his behalf. He has the right to know, by name, the physician responsible for coordinating his care.

3.   The patient **has the right to receive from his physician information necessary to give informed consent prior**[2] to the start of any procedure and/or treatment. Except in emergencies, such information for informed consent should include, but not necessarily be limited to the specific procedure and/or treatment, the **medically significant risks involved** and the probable duration of the incapacitation. Where medically significant alternatives for care or treatment exist, or **when the patient requests information concerning medical alternatives, the patient has the right to such information.**[3] The patient also has the right to know the name of the person responsible for the procedures and/or treatment.

4.   The patient has the right to **refuse treatment to the extent**[4] permitted by law and to be informed of the medical consequences of his action.

5.   The patient has the right to every consideration of his privacy concerning his own medical care program. Case discussion, consultation, examination, and treatment are confidential and should be conducted discreetly. **Those not directly involved in his care must have the permission of the patient to be present.**[5]

6.   The patient has the right to expect that all communications and records pertaining to his care should be treated as confidential.

7.   The patient has the right to expect that within its capacity a hospital must make reasonable response to the request of a patient for services. The hospital must provide evaluation, service, and/or referral as indicated by the urgency of the case. When medically permissible, a patient may be transferred to another facility only after he has received complete information and explanation concerning the needs for and alternative to such a transfer. The institution to which the patient is to be transferred must first have accepted the patient for transfer.

8.   The patient has the right to **obtain any information as to any relationship of his hospital to other health care and educational institutions insofar as his care is concerned.** The patient has the right to obtain information as to the **existence of any professional relationships among individuals,**[6] by name, who are treating him.

9.   The patient has the right to be advised if the hospital proposes to engage in or **perform human experimentation affecting his care or treatment.**[7] The patient has the right to refuse to participate in such research projects.

10.   The patient has the right to expect reasonable continuity of care. He has the right to know in advance what appointment times and physicians are available and where. The patient has the right to expect that the hospital will provide a mechanism whereby he is informed by his physician or a delegate of the physician of the patient's continuing health care requirements following discharge.

11.   The patient has the **right to examine and receive an explanation of his bill**[8] regardless of source of payment.

12.   The patient has the right to know what hospital rules and regulations apply to his conduct as a patient.

No catalog of rights can guarantee for the patient the kind of treatment he has a right to expect. A hospital has many functions to perform, including the prevention and treatment of disease, the education of both health professionals and patients, and the conduct of clinical research. All these activities must be conducted with an overriding concern for the patient and, above all, the recognition of his dignity as a human being. Success in achieving this recognition assures success in the defense of the rights of the patient.

Approved by the American Hospital Association   February 6, 1973

Opening
Paragraph

A.   This statement indicates that patients should consider themselves as equal partners with the physician in the treatment plan. And that you should not consider yourselves subordinate as you share the responsibility for your own healthcare.

B.   It is important in the treatment of your medical condition that you provide as much detailed information about your medical condition and your past medical treatment.

C.   Both the physician and the patient should be comfortable with each other and develop a mutual respect.

Statement

1A.   You have the right to receive all the information you require concerning the benefits, risks and costs of your treatment.

1B.   You may receive copies of your medical records. While some states specifically do not allow this, most physicians will provide copies if asked.

1C.   Patients have the right to have their questions answered and AMA Medical Ethics reinforce this by stating that the questions must be answered honestly.

1D.   This indicates that the physician should voluntarily advise the patient of any potential conflicts of interest (*i.e.,* ownership of labs or sharing of profits in the group practice with other specialties to who you may be referred).

2A.   You have the right to follow or not follow the advice of your physician.

5A.   The physician may not discontinue your treatment plan without giving you time to seek another doctor.

6A.   Physicians should occasionally provide free or discounted medical treatment.

Fundamental Elements of the Patient-Physician Relationship

The following report of the Council on Ethical and Judicial Affairs was adopted by the AMA House of Delegates on June 26, 1990.

From ancient times, physicians have recognized that the health and well-being of patients depends on a collaborative effort between physician and patient. *Patients share with physicians the responsibility for their own health care.[A]* The patient-physician relationship is of greatest benefit to patients when they bring medical problems to the attention of their physicians in a timely fashion, *provide information about their medical condition* to the *best of their ability,[B]* and work with their physicians in a *mutually respectful alliance.[C]* Physicians can best contribute to this alliance by serving as their patients' advocate and by fostering the following rights:

1. The patient has the right to *receive information from physicians* and to *discuss the benefits, risks, and costs of appropriate treatment alternatives.[1A]* Patients should receive guidance from their physicians as to the optimal course of action. Patients are also entitled to *obtain copies* or summaries of their *medical records,[1B]* to have *their questions answered,[1C]* to be advised of *potential conflicts of interest[1D]* that their physicians might have, and to receive independent professional opinions.

2. The patient has the right to make decisions regarding the health care that is recommended by his or her physician. Accordingly, *patients may accept or refuse any recommended medical treatment.[2A]*

3. The patient has the right to courtesy, respect, dignity, responsiveness, and timely attention to his or her needs.

4. The patient has the right to confidentiality. The physician should not reveal confidential communications or information without the consent of the patient, unless provided for by law or by the need to protect the welfare of the individual or the public interest.

5. The patient has the right to continuity of health care. The physician has an obligation to cooperate in the coordination of medically indicated care with other health care providers treating the patient. The physician *may not discontinue treatment of a patient* as long as further treatment is medically indicated, without giving the patient *sufficient opportunity to make alternative arrangements for care.[5A]*

6. The patient has a basic right to have available adequate health care. Physicians, along with the rest of society, should continue to work toward this goal. Fulfillment of this right is dependent on society providing resources so that no patient is deprived of necessary care because of an inability to pay for the care. *Physicians should continue their traditional assumption of a part of the responsibility for the medical care of those who cannot afford essential health care[6A].*

Readings About Consent

If the reader would like more detailed information about the informed consent process, the following books are suggested. These are specialty books and may not be available at your local library or bookstore. We found these in a college law library.

Consent to Treatment — A Practical Guide 2nd Edition, 1990
    Fay A. Rozovsky, J.D., M.P.H.
    Little, Brown & Company

Informed Consent — A Guide for Health Care Providers, 1981
    Arnold J. Rosoff
    An Aspen Publication

Informed Consent — Legal Theory and Clinical Practice, 1987
    Appelbaum, Lidz, Meisel
    Oxford University Press, Inc.

Hospital Liability — Law and Practice, 5th Edition, 1987
    Bertolet and Goldsmith
    Practicing Law Institute

Hospital Liability, 1990
    Law Journal Seminars Press

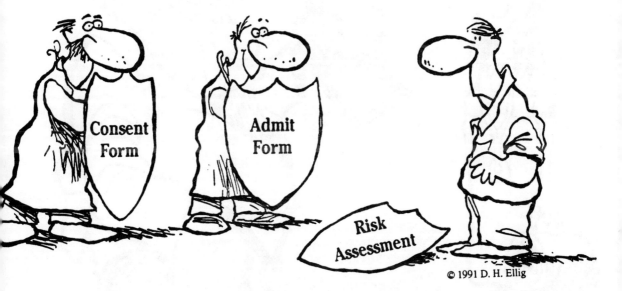

© 1991 D. H. Ellig

Pick Up Your Shield

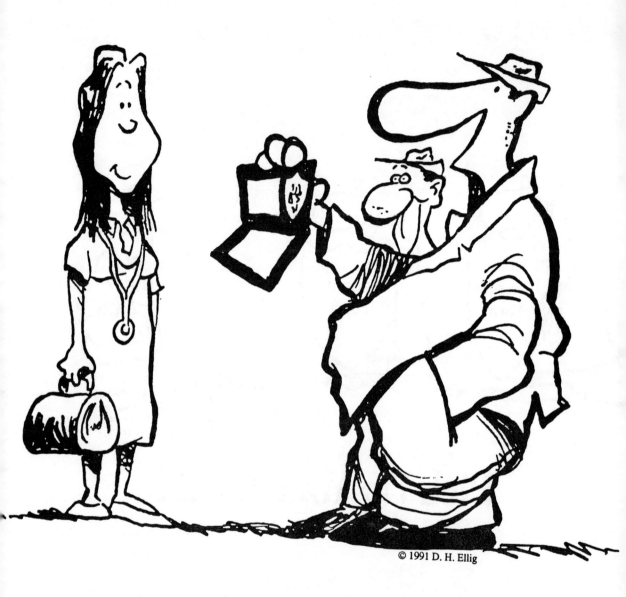

© 1991 D. H. Ellig

Just The Facts Ma'am

CHAPTER 6

ASK YOUR DOCTOR

INTRODUCTION

Most healthcare consumers spend more time qualifying the sales person of their new TV than they do qualifying their healthcare provider. The healthcare provider will be treating your most *precious possession, your child or spouse.* Yet we spend less then qualifying the healthcare provider than we do the salesperson. *It doesn't make sense.*

The following are suggested topics that may be helpful when discussing your treatment plan with your physician. Do not be afraid to ask questions. An easy, non-threatening way to ask questions is to start your questions with, "Tell me about . . . ." The healthcare consumer is given the right to ask questions and doctors are required to give honest answers by the Informed Consent Doctrine and AMA Ethics. The questions in this chapter are a starting point for opening the physician/patient dialogue and are merely suggestions

Request specific answers to questions, not general responses. If possible, get answers in simple, non-medical terms. For example, how many people out of 100 have successes, complications or failures? Ask to see documented studies on which the doctor is basing his recommendations.

Healthcare is changing so rapidly that to expect your doctor to know the latest research and studies of all the conditions they treat plus be aware of all the new drugs and their complications is putting too much of a burden on them. They simply don't have time to read all the journals! But you can research your condition and should. If you want to do your own research, see Chapter 8 on computer access of the most recent studies and articles about your condition or treatment.

Take a Friend, Take Notes, or Take A Recorder!!!

As unusual as it may seem to record your conversation with your doctor, you may find that your doctor is recording the discussion. The reason some doctors now record doctor/patient discussions is to provide an excellent source of reference. Some medical malpractice insurance company's risk management services recommend that doctors record doctor/patient conversations to provide a complete record. In the past, some doctors' file notes lacked important data necessary to defend doctors from medical malpractice claims.

One of the common problems patients encounter in discussing treatment is the physician's use of technical medical terms which are difficult for the patient to understand. Physicians use medical jargon to describe *what* the illness or condition is and *how* they will treat it. What we need are more bilingual doctors, doctors who can speak medical jargon with colleagues, hospitals and insurance companies and simple English with simple probabilities for patients. The patient doesn't need to know *how* the procedure is done. They don't ask the automobile mechanic how he is going to change the water pump and the mechanic doesn't tell them how he is going to do it. They just know that it will be fixed and the odds are high that it will fix the problem. Patient concerns are very simple and the answers can also be very simple.

The patient really only wants to know:

Question	Doctor Response
What do I have?	Medical jargon okay — simple answer better
Can you fix it?	Yes / no / maybe
What are the chances your fix will work?	_____%
What are the risks of the fix?	Complications _____%
	Disability _____%
	Death _____%
	Drug Side Effects — simple feeling terms
What if I don't get it fixed?	It will go away — yes / no
	It will get worse — yes / no

The patient's main concerns can be simply quantified. Most patients can understand probabilities, since they deal with probabilities every day.

Remember,

"There is nothing so complex that cannot be explained simply."

— Albert Einstein

A patient can not legally give informed consent for treatment unless he understands the treatment and its risks. It is the doctor's responsibility to explain the treatment in terms the patient can understand. **The audience cannot be faulted if it doesn't understand the speaker.**

It is the patient's responsibility to understand the doctor. If you submit to treatment it will be assumed that you understood all the risks of treatment and its expected outcome. If you don't understand, tell the doctor or he can only assume you understand.

Doctor As Your Guide

Think of your doctor as your tour guide through the medical services industry system. He has the primary responsibility for your care as you move from healthcare provider to healthcare provider. He should be able to help you get the information suggested in this book. If you encounter difficulties receiving answers from other medical providers to the suggested questions, it is entirely proper for you to ask your doctor for help in getting this information. He is responsible for referring you to other medical providers and has AMA Ethic Guidelines (see Appendix) to know the quality of the providers to which he has referred you.

If you experience difficulties obtaining mortality rates, infection rates, number of times your procedure has been performed, complication rates, or other matters, ask your referring doctor to get this information for you.

If the referred doctor does not care to address questions about the number of times he has performed the procedure, his cost, or any of the other questions addressed in this book, ask your referring doctor for his help.

If the lab is hesitant to provide you accuracy information about the testing procedures, ask your referring doctor to get this information.

Your surgeon selects a hospital and assembles a team of anesthesiologists, radiologists and pathologists. If any of these individuals have difficulty responding to your qualifying or cost questions, ask your surgeon for help.

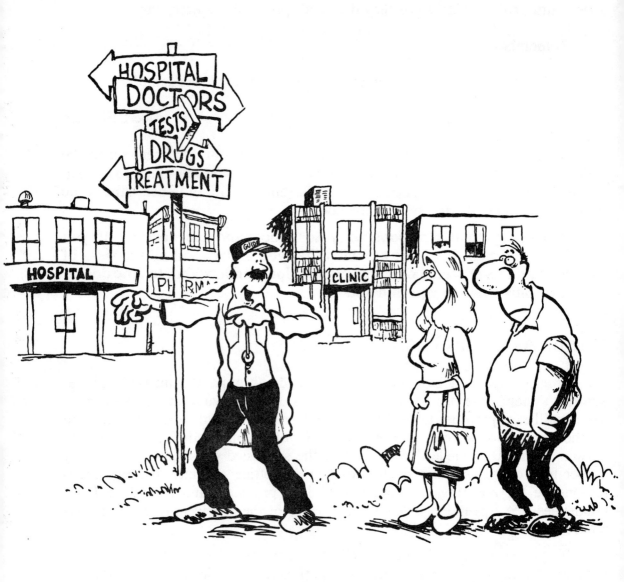

Reading the suggested questions, you may think, "I can't ask my doctor these questions. He'll get upset and he's the person who's going to operate on me. I don't want him upset." This is a concern expressed by many people. If the patient really feels that the doctor could be that vicious, demented and twisted to change the quality of treatment because of questions asked, then the patient **better** find another doctor.

The questions are suggested for *your* benefit, so that you become fully informed of your treatment and your doctor's expectations. In our society, the doctor is viewed at the *highest level of professionalism* and, therefore, we should expect the *highest level of professionalism in response* to our questions. By law and AMA Ethics, doctors are required to answer patients' questions honestly. Doctors are therefore obligated to answer questions when asked. If you do not receive this high level of professionalism in response to your questions, you may want to factor this lack of response into your decision concerning the use of this doctor. It is extremely important that you have a comfortable doctor/patient relationship.

Your stake in the treatment is greater than the doctor's. The doctor's ego and reputation are on the line, but it may be your life or the quality of your life after treatment that is on the line for you. *Your interest is greater than the doctor's.*

****

CONCEPT AT WORK:

First Story — An individual covered by an HMO took his child to the primary care physician. The daughter's stomach problems required surgery and the primary care physician said he would perform the surgery. The father asked about the primary care physician's qualifications to perform this operation, such as special training, number of times performed, and other quality issues. At this point the primary care physician recommended a surgeon. The father asked the same questions of the surgeon and then insisted on a pediatric surgeon.

During the surgery it was discovered that the 10-month old's condition was much worse and more complicated than anticipated and that the experience of the pediatric surgeon was necessary. The surgery went well, the child recovered and is doing fine.

Second Story — An individual requiring surgery asked all the doctors if they would waive any excess fees (accept only what the insurance company considered "reasonable"). All the doctors agreed and the patient didn't have to pay $12,000 in excessive fees.

****

Some of the questions addressed in the following sections are also documented on the Risk Assessment Form for your convenience in the chapter *"What You Should Really Be Told."*

In today's mobile society, very few of us have a long-term relationship with any one physician. Many of us have been in the position of arriving in a new location and having to find a new physician.

This chapter will help you qualify your new physician.

Finding a new physician in a new location is always difficult. The following sources however, are a good place to start:

Local medical society
Hospital referral services (a marketing service for doctors who practice at
    that hospital)
Ask a nurse
Ask friends or business associates
Ask people in a local support group

When you call the medical society, hospitals or support groups you may be able to do some preliminary qualifying using the questions in this chapter.

QUESTIONS FOR ALL DOCTORS

Many times doctors are faulted for being very quick with patients and not appearing to give their full attention. The next time you meet your doctor try smiling and provide a happy greeting. All day long doctors are meeting worried, concerned patients. It's no wonder that they adopt the attitudes of their patients. If you try a smile and happy face, you will probably get a happy face in return. More importantly, you will have started to establish a relationship of equal partners rather than doctor/body in need of repair.

Put In Writing?

*   Will you put your treatment plan, expectations and risks in writing?

Placing expectations and risks in writing *before* treatment will not only clarify any misunderstandings or communication problems, but will also provide an excellent reference source after treatment.

As we all know from personal and business transactions, *"the palest ink is better than the best memory."* Items and issues placed in writing tend to be well thought through and more conservative than verbal statements. We all know this from other personal and business transactions.

If the doctor refuses to put his treatment plans in writing, you might consider putting your written understanding of the treatment or surgery in a letter to your doctor using the Risk Assessment Form described in the chapter on Consent Forms. You should conclude by asking his agreement on your understanding and response before treatment.

How Much?

* How much will the treatment cost?

    This is an important question. Many people have seen their insurance deductible increase (from $50 in 1980 to $250 in 1990), and as a result most of us now have to pay for the first visit. Of course, if you have no insurance or a very high deductible ($1,000), you will be responsible for all the cost.

    Remember to ask for the cost of an initial visit, because the doctor will charge more for the first visit since they must spend time taking a medical history. Also ask what the charge is for a return visit. It should be less.

    Tell the staff you want the lowest Medicare or managed care price.

* Will you quote prices before treatment is provided?

    Without price, the patient cannot make a value judgement. Knowing the price before treatment will also eliminate any surprises. Medical treatment can be very expensive even when very little time is involved. It is possible to run up a bill of $250/$300 in 15 minutes. Just because the bill is $250/$300 for 15 minutes work, doesn't mean the patient doesn't have to pay.

    If we don't ask about prices how can we be upset when the bill arrives? We have given the provider the opportunity to charge whatever they want, with no negotiation or value judgment on our part.

    When we enter into a contract for services without knowing price we are setting ourselves up for a rude awakening when the bill arrives. It is best to get a **price first** or at least an estimate of services.

Waive Excess Fees?

* If your charges exceed the insurance "reasonable fee," will you waive the excess?

    For most patients "will you waive excess fees" are probably the most important five words in this entire book. It is imperative that you settle the cost issue with your doctor before treatment in the event your insurance company denies full payment because of an "unreasonable fee." It is much easier to negotiate a charge reduction before services are rendered than later when the bill collectors are at your door.

    A great many doctors will respond positively to this question. If your doctor doesn't, you might want to consider this factor in your medical care selection process. The *AMA Principles of Medical Ethics* states that a physician should not charge or collect excessive fees. Reasonable fees are determined by a person knowledgeable as to current fees (an insurance company?).

If surgery is to be performed, you should also inquire about the appropriateness of the assistant surgeon's fees. A common complaint of patients who have had surgery is that the assistant surgeon's charges were not covered because the insurance company stated that the use of an assistant surgeon was not appropriate.

If the patient does not address the assistant surgeon fees now, he may have to pay a portion or all of the fees later. In most cases, the patient won't even know who the assistant surgeon was until he gets the bill. This is a good reason to use the cost estimator form at the end of this chapter. It will reveal most of the charges the patient might incur.

PPO Doctor

*   Are you a preferred or participating doctor?
*   Will you refer only to other preferred providers?

If your doctor is a member of your insurance company's preferred provider organization (PPO) or a participating doctor with Medicare or Blue Cross Blue Shield plans, the physician is not allowed to collect excess billed amounts from the patient.

These doctors have signed an agreement with the insurance companies stating they will accept a predetermined amount and cannot collect any more from the patient. Occasionally the physician's office staff or billing service will attempt to collect these excess amounts. If this happens, explain that you are not responsible for the excess payments and report the activity to your insurance company.

The second question is important because if your doctor refers you to non-preferred providers you will be responsible for more cost. Therefore, you should expect your doctor to help you control cost by referring you only to other preferred providers. Unfortunately it is quite common for doctors to refer to non-preferred providers such as a non-preferred x-ray lab and radiologist. See Chapter 15, "Watch Out For The Bill," which will give you some ideas on how to handle non-preferred provider bills with excessive charges.

Access to Medical Records

*   Will you provide me with copies of my medical records?

As of early 1990, 26 states had laws which gave patients the right to receive their own medical records.

Medical records provide doctors with relevant information about the patient's medical past treatments, conditions, and allergies which help the doctor treat the patient. It would seem that most doctors would want the patient to have access to his past medical history, so the patient can be treated with the least amount of risk. A written medical record would appear to be a more reliable source of medical data than patient memory.

How would you react if the contractor who worked on your house or the auto mechanic who fixed your car refused to provide you written documentation (the blue prints of the house) of what they did or what wrong they fixed? Why does the patient willingly accept the fact that he cannot access his own medical records?

Why do you suppose patients cannot access their records in some states? Who is protected by the lack of patient access to his own medical records: the patient or the physician?

If your doctor refuses to provide you with your medical records, place your request in writing, reiterating his refusal. In your letter, indicate the date of the refusal and your willingness to pay for the cost of copying, and also request that the medical records be provided by a certain date.

The good news is that a survey of physicians showed that nearly 75 percent had no objection to releasing records to their patients even in those states that restrict patient access.

Date _____

To Whom It May Concern:

I hereby agree to release the patient's medical and hospital records to the patient if the patient so requests. Please honor their request.

This patient also wants to be informed of all treatment information to include test results, reason for tests, drug information and treatment results.

The patient may be responsible for a copy charge of ____ per sheet.

This agreement is in effect for one (1) year from the date of this letter.

_____   _____
Patient   Doctor

Take this letter to the hospital, without this letter the hospital may refuse your request for your medical records.

If you would like more information about access to medical records the following are good sources:

American Medical Records Association
919 N. Michigan Ave., Suite 1400
Chicago, IL 60611

Request the free brochure "Your Health Information Belongs to You" with a self-addressed, stamped business envelope.

Health Research Group, Publications Manager
2000 P Street NW, Suite 700
Washington, DC 20036

Request a copy of the booklet "Medical Records: Getting Yours." This booklet costs $5.00.

MIB Information Office
P.O. Box 105, Essex Station
Boston, MA 02112

Through this organization you may request a copy of the medical information they have on file. MIB operates much like credit bureaus that are used by banks to check your credit history. MIB is a medical history bureau used by the insurance industry to check your medical history.

If you review your medical records and find errors you may request a correction.

Medical Society Member

*   Is your doctor a member of the local medical society?

This is important if you ever have a future dispute with your doctor. If the doctor is not a member of the local medical society your request for "peer review" cannot be administrated by the local medical society and you will have to register your complaint with the state board of medical examiners.

Physician's Assistants and Nurse Practitioners

*   Does the doctor's staff include physician's assistants (PA's) and nurse practitioners (NP's)?

Physician's assistants and nurse practitioners are normally licensed to perform medical work which is more advanced than the nursing staff can provide but less than what the physician can provide. They can normally diagnose and treat the more common conditions and illnesses and provide follow-up treatment based on the physician's instructions.

A physician's office that uses nurse practitioners and physician's assistants normally means that the office will work more efficiently. The physician can use his time and training more effectively on the more serious cases. It also should result in less costly treatment, since the fees for a nurse practitioner and physician's assistant should be less than the physician.

Despite the economics and efficiencies of using physician's assistants and nurse practitioners, it is interesting to note that they are far fewer in number than physicians. Not many physicians use physician's assistants and nurse practitioners.

For Females

*   Will the doctor have a nurse present during examinations?

Occasionally there have been newspaper reports of male doctors molesting female patients. As a result most male doctors now have female nurses present during examinations. This provides protection both for the physician and for the patient. The physician is protected from unwarranted harassment suits and the patient is protected from actual harassment.

Life Prolonging Issues

*   What are your views on life prolonging issues?

It is important that you discuss with your physician his feelings on life prolonging issues, particularly as they relate to terminal or comatose patients. It is important that both the patient and the physician have common views on this issue. The patient may want to provide the physician with a copy of his Living Will instructions as outlined in our chapter on that subject.

QUESTIONS FOR THE PRIMARY CARE DOCTOR

Follow-up Visits

*   Do I *really* have to return for a follow-up visit? How much will it cost?

    Why not see if you can simply call in your condition or treatment results.

Phone Access

*   Will you offer advice or renew prescriptions over the phone?

    In the rapidly changing health services field, some physicians are now willing to do this. It is particularly common among doctors who are paid a monthly (capitation) fee to provide all necessary treatment for each patient enrolled with the insurance company. This type of payment means the doctor does not have to see a patient to get paid by the insurance company. The doctor is paid whether he treats the patient or not. Some doctors change their office philosophy based on their reimbursement arrangement with the insurance company.

Waiting Time

*   What is your average waiting time? If my waiting time is longer, will you compensate me for my excessive waiting time?

    Why not call before leaving the house or office to confirm your appointment time?

Specialist Referral

*   Why must I see a specialist? Why this type of specialist? Is this particular specialist part of your group practice or a friend?

    NOW IS THE TIME TO TAKE CHARGE! Most doctors will provide only one name as a referral, ask for three names and their qualifications. With three names you can exercise some control, as you will make the decision on who will treat you.

    The purpose of this question is to ensure that you are referred to the most qualified specialist and not just because the specialist is a member of the physician's group practice who may share revenue or who is a personal friend.

QUESTIONS IF REFERRED TO A SPECIALIST

Board Certified

* Are you Board Certified (not just Board Qualified)?

As doctors narrow their field of interest they receive designations that show they have received more training and studies in their area of interest. Two important designations are Board Certified Specialist and Fellowship.

BOARD QUALIFIED — All doctors are board qualified if they have graduated from a medical school and have completed residency.

BOARD CERTIFIED — This is a doctor who has graduated from medical school, had residency in a specialty and passed a written and oral exam to validate his knowledge in the specialty. Normally, additional studies are required to pass the examination; therefore it may be appropriate to consider a board certified physician to be slightly more knowledgeable. It should not be necessarily interpreted that *all* board certified physicians are better than all non-board certified ones. However, studies have shown that outcomes by Board Certified doctors as a group are more successful than non board certified.

Of course you will want the board certification to be in the specialty procedure or treatment you require. Just because a doctor is board certified in one area does not mean that he is board certified or knowledgeable in all areas.

As healthcare consumers have gotten smarter, they are more and more seeking the services of a Board Certified Specialist. In response to consumer demand, more and more doctors have become "Board Certified." *A word of caution.* There are approximately 140 specialty boards, some of which are "self-designated" boards and not recognized by the AMA. Some "self-designated" may have only minimal membership standards, such as a fee, no residency training and only a simple test to join. It is important that your specialist have extensive training with the procedure to be performed.

****

CONCEPT AT WORK:

Recently the media reported the case of a woman who went to a "Board Certified Plastic Surgeon" for a breast uplift and received a breast augmentation because the "Board Certified" doctor did not know how to do an uplift. The family practice doctor had become a "Board Certified Plastic Surgeon" because he had done "x" number of chemical face peels, passed a simple written test and paid a membership fee. It allowed the doctor to post a degree that said "Board Certified Plastic Surgeon" when the doctor had *never* done a plastic surgery procedure below the neck.

Result for the patient: embarrassment, a whole new wardrobe and having to save $5,800 for another surgery — breast reduction. Malpractice insurance did not cover the breast surgery, because the insurance company would not cover plastic surgery performed by a family practice doctor with insufficient experience.

****

A specialist certified by the American Board of Medical Specialist (ABMS) has generally had the most complete training and testing. You may call 800-776-2378 for a list of ABMS doctors in your area. The ABMS program is recognized by the AMA.

The list below shows some of the specialty areas certified by the American Board of Medical Specialties (ABMS). There are also *subspecialty certifications* within each of these specialties.

Diplomate American Board of **Allergy and Immunology**	D.A.I.
Diplomate American Board of **Anesthesiology**	D.A.
Diplomate American Board of **Colon and Rectal Surgery**	D.CR.
Diplomate American Board of **Dermatology**	D.D.
Diplomate American Board of **Emergency Medicine**	D.EM.
Diplomate American Board of **Family Practice**	D.F.P.
Diplomate American Board of **Internal Medicine**	D.IM.
Diplomate American Board of **Neurological Surgery**	D.NS.
Diplomate American Board of **Nuclear Medicine**	D.NM.
Diplomate American Board of **Ophthalmology**	D.O.
Diplomate American Board of **Obstetrics and Gynecology**	D.OG.
Diplomate American Board of **Otolaryngology**	D.OL.
Diplomate American Board of **Orthopedic Surgery**	D.OS.
Diplomate American Board of **Pathology**	D.PA.
Diplomate American Board of **Pediatrics**	D.P.
Diplomate American Board of **Preventive Medicine**	D.PM.
Diplomate American Board of **Physical Medicine and Rehabilitation**	D.PMR.
Diplomate American Board of **Psychiatry and Neurology**	D.PN.

Diplomate American Board of Plastic Surgery	D.PS.
Diplomate American Board of Radiology	D.R.
Diplomate American Board of Surgery	D.S.
Diplomate of the Board of Thoracic Surgery	D.TS.
Diplomate American Board of Urology	D.U.

If you do not want to use the ABMS toll free number you may use the *Directory of Medical Specialists* at your local library. This book lists all the physicians who have been board certified and also indicates their credentials.

It is interesting to note that only 163,000 of 500,000 doctors in the United States are not certified as specialists. The United States has more specialists than any country in the world, but we lack primary care physicians. The rest of the world lacks specialists.

FELLOWSHIP — Is an additional recognition conferred by a group of specialists on one of their members in recognition of outstanding work, study or significant contribution to their field of study. It normally indicates that the fellow is well qualified to practice the specialty due to education, training and experience. As an example, a physician that has the letters F.A.C.S. after M.D. means not only is he a specialist in surgery but also a member of the American College of Surgeons.

Below is a list of fellowship initials that may follow M.D.:

A.F.A.C.A.L.	Allergists	Associate Fellow of American College of Allergists
F.A.A.P.	Pediatrics	Fellow American Academy of Pediatrics
F.A.C.A.L.	Allergists	Fellow of American College of Allergists
F.A.C.A.	Angiology	Fellow of American College of Angiology
F.A.C.A.n.	Anesthesiology	Fellow of American College of Anesthesiologists
F.A.C.C.	Cardiologists	Fellow of American College of Cardiology
F.C.C.P.	Chest Physicians	Fellow of American College of Chest Physicians
F.A.C.G.	Gastroenterologists	Fellow of American College of Gastroenterology
F.A.C.O.G.	OB/GYN	Fellow of American College of Obstetricians and Gynecologists
F.C.A.P.	Pathologists	Fellow of College of American Pathologists
F.A.C.P.	Physicians	Fellow of American College of Physicians
F.A.C.P.M.	Preventive Medicine	Fellow of American College of Preventive Medicine
F.A.C.R.	Radiologists	Fellow of American College of Radiology
F.A.C.S.	Surgeons	Fellow of American College of Surgeons
F.I.C.S.	Surgeons	Fellow of International College of Surgeons

The *Medical Association Directory of Physicians* lists all doctors in the United States and is available at the library. If your doctor is not listed it may be appropriate to ask him why. The most common reason for not being listed is a recent graduation. If your doctor is not listed you should ask why and check carefully.

Doctor's Experience

*   How often have you performed this procedure?

Numerous studies indicate that success rates increase dramatically with the number of times a physician performs the procedure. You should expect 40 to 50 a year, one per week to maintain proficiency. *The average surgeon performs approximately 200 surgeries per year. That means one-half perform less than 200; you may want the surgeons in the top half. But remember that is 200 surgeries not necessarily 200 of the procedure you need. So ask about* **your procedure.**

We realize that every physician must perform a new procedure on a patient for the first time, but if we have a choice, we may not want to be the first patient.

Doctors who develop new surgical procedures and their peers establish guidelines indicating training and experience necessary for performing a new surgical procedure safely.

Normally training follows guidelines such as:

Attend "how to" seminars
Observe X number of operations
Assist X number of operations
Operate with teacher X number of operations*
Finally qualified to operate solo

*   Refer to Chapter No. 5 to learn how to ensure only the doctor you interviewed performs your surgery.

A sample of this additional training is suggested by the American College of Cardiology guidelines for performance of an angioplasty (a surgical procedure in which a balloon or laser is inserted to remove blockage in an artery). The guidelines suggest these steps before a surgeon is qualified to perform the angioplasty on a solo basis.

Observe experts
Attend "how to" seminars
Three years of specialty training
Plus one additional year
Involved with 125 procedures (75 as primary doctor)
Continue with one procedure per week (52 per year)

The above guidelines are very strict and intensive. Few doctors can meet this guideline. How many doctors in your community who perform angioplasties can meet these guidelines? How many hospitals? It is simple to check the physician's experience, just ask and record the information on your informed consent check list.

* What is your success rate? What is your definition of success?

Occasionally a doctor's definition of success may differ greatly from a patient's expectations for success. This can and does lead to doctor/patient disputes.

The American College of Cardiology guidelines for a successful angioplasty is to reduce the blockage 20 percent or more. The patient may expect a total removal of the blockage, in which case the doctor will consider a 50 percent change a success and the patient will consider it a failure.

Complete discussion of what is a success will improve the doctor/patient relationship. If the doctor had said 70 percent to 80 percent of the operations are successful (producing a 20 percent improvement), and the patient thought success was total removal, it could result in a very serious dispute and loss of patient faith in their doctor.

Patient References

* May I have the name of one or two patients who have had this surgery?

With almost any other product or service we ask for satisfied customer references. Yet, we feel uncomfortable asking our physicians this question.

Former patients make excellent sources for treatment plan success, feelings during recovery, doctor/patient relationship information, and, most importantly, did they return to same the lifestyle activities as before and how soon. Since former patients are such excellent resources of information, and support groups are made up of individuals currently undergoing treatment or having treatment in the past, they are an excellent source of information. Please refer to the chapter on support groups to find out which groups are available and how to contact them.

It is very common for physicians to deny patient referrals due to "doctor/patient confidentiality." If this reference is important to you, you might suggest that the doctor call several former patients to see if they will discuss their surgery with you. Doctors, of course, can get a release from all patients the same as when they get a release stating your medical records may be released to insurance companies and other doctors.

Physician surveys have indicated that only one in ten physicians will give patient referrals. As a result, it may be difficult for you to get patient referrals from the doctor. You may want to use the help of the support groups of people who are currently in treatment or who have had treatment.

Fees

* How much is your fee for the surgery and follow-up visits?

* How much will the hospital cost? Can the procedure be done on an outpatient basis?

Estimated Bill

* Can I have a sample bill for your anticipated services?

    Ask your doctor to produce a sample bill from his computerized billing system noting all the services he anticipates providing for your treatment.

    This should be a simple task for most physicians. If the physician can't provide an estimated bill because he doesn't know what will be done or what will be found, the patient may want the physician to provide a more definitive response, rather than a "hunting expedition."

Outpatient Treatment

* Will this procedure be done on an outpatient basis?

    If this procedure is to be done on an outpatient basis, you will want to know if the doctor can also perform the procedure in the hospital. If the hospital has not admitted the doctor to perform the procedure on an inpatient basis, you probably don't want the doctor to do the procedure, since the hospital has not qualified the doctor for this procedure.

    If surgery is to be done on an outpatient basis you should also qualify the facility.

Is it accredited by the American Association for Accreditation of Ambulatory Centers?

Does it have cardiorespiratory equipment?

Is staff qualified to use equipment?

Who will administer and monitor anesthesia?

A Certified Registered Nurse Anesthetist?

What arrangements have been made with the nearest hospital in case of emergency?

Outpatient surgery has become popular in recent years because it originally was very cost efficient (100 percent paid and no deductible). The healthcare market has reacted to the demand and now outpatient surgery may be more expensive than in-hospital treatment.

If you are concerned about cost you may want to check what the same procedure would cost in the hospital or at a **non-hospital affiliated** outpatient facility.

Don't forget you can generally get cost estimates by asking for a copy of a previous bill from the provider.

Anesthesiologist Referral

* Why have you selected this particular anesthesiologist?

Your referring physician's response to this question is very important, since the anesthesiologist is probably the second most important member of the surgery team. You should ask: How many times have you used this anesthesiologist? How long has he practiced? Has he been referred to the Board of Medical Examiners? Is he certified substance abuse free?

Often we do not meet our anesthesiologist until he is ready to perform his service. Now is the time to discuss the qualifications of the anesthesiologist. Once you're on the operating table, it is too late.

QUESTIONS ABOUT YOUR TREATMENT

Diagnosis

* When a clear diagnosis can't be made, will doctor admit it?

* What are the possibilities of a misdiagnosis of my condition?

This question directly addresses the "infallibility" issue of doctors. The benefit of asking this question is that the patient becomes aware that occasionally the doctor can be unsure of the diagnosis. It serves to remind the doctor that there is always a possibility of error because of testing or incomplete data. And it reminds the physician of past diagnosis mistakes.

Be extremely cautious if the response is never, unless you are eight months pregnant or having a limb or digit replaced. Most physicians should admit to occasional misdiagnosis depending on the condition.

Misdiagnosis or failure to diagnose is one of the major causes of doctor/patient litigation, which would indicate that occasionally physicians do misdiagnose or fail to diagnose.

Be sure you learn how to spell your diagnosis so that you may do your own research at your home medical library or with computer retrieval of recent studies as discussed later.

Risks

*   What are the risks associated with this procedure?

After the patient knows what illness or condition he has and how it can be treated, the next issue he wants to know is how risky is this procedure. Risk includes the chances for success, chances for failure, chances for complications and the risks to life and lifestyle.

The physician should be able to put the answers to these questions in very simple terms based on odds. This should not be a hard question to answer, but some physicians may slip into medical jargon. Don't let them — you want odds!

Be sure you know how to spell the suggested procedure and alternatives so you can research the latest medical studies as discussed in Chapter 8.

If the physician has treated your condition before, he knows what the odds and risks are. The physician is legally bound to tell you these facts before you can give informed consent. In rare incidents he may withhold risk information from the patient if the physician feels it will cause the patient distress and harm the treatment process. But he must give this information to someone associated with the patient. This is the basis of informed consent.

Invasive surgery (a procedure that penetrates the skin) increases risk dramatically. The malpractice table reflects a 310 percent premium difference for a family doctor who performs invasive surgery and one who doesn't. This would seem to indicate that there are risks with invasive surgery, **be sure you understand them.**

The table also shows that medical malpractice is not nearly as expensive as we have been lead to believe for a majority of doctors. In Arizona only 3 percent of doctors perform thoracic surgery or neurosurgery which have the highest rates.

Specialty	Annual Malpractice Premium
Family Practice (no surgery)	$ 9,000*
Internal Medicine	$ 9,000
Ophthalmology	$ 9,000
Radiology	$ 9,000
Pediatrics	$11,000
Urology	$13,000
Family Practice (minor surgery)	$15,000
Neurology	$15,000
Radiology (interventional)	$15,000
Emergency Medicine	$18,000
Internal Medicine (angiography)	$21,000
Internal Medicine (interventional)	$21,000
Family Practice (with surgery)	$28,000*
Plastic Surgery	$28,000
Anesthesia	$31,000
General Surgery	$31,000
Otolaryngology	$31,000
Orthopedic Surgery	$35,000
Thoracic Surgery (without pump)	$35,000
OB/GYN	$51,000
Thoracic Surgery (with pump)	$59,000
Neurosurgery	$71,000

$10,730 was the average malpractice insurance for all doctors in 1989. This was 4.2 percent of their gross revenue. Since then malpractice premiums have gone down.

Complications

* What complications *might* occur — infections, anaesthesia, reactions?
* How long before I will be able to resume normal activities?

You might want to have complications information placed in writing and documented along with studies upon which the doctor is basing his decision. This information in written form will ensure that you and your doctor understand the outcome, the success and the limits of his suggested treatment plan.

*   What are the complications that may occur from this surgery?

It is very difficult for doctors to talk about three subjects; price, risk and complications. We have addressed the first two and now will provide some help on how to address the issue of complications.

The complications that may occur from surgery are:

Infections	Anesthesia
Adhesions	Drug Therapy
Hemorrhaging	Implant Device Rejection
Scarring	Procedure Risk

Infections — The most common complication of surgery is a nosocomial (hospital acquired infection). You should ask the doctor what the probability of a hospital acquired infection is (normally about 10 percent) and what he will do to reduce it.

Adhesions are when injured tissue adhere (grow together) and usually occur with internal organs and tissue and often require a *second surgery* to correct. The most common site is in the abdomenal area.

Hemorrhage — This is medical jargon for bleeding and if it is noticed after surgery may require a *second surgery* to stop the bleeding.

Scarring normally refers to injured exterior tissue and you may ask your physician how he intends to keep the scarring to a minimum.

Anesthesia — Ask the physician about the complication of anesthesia and also inform him of any previous reactions and that you would like the anesthesia with the least risk.

Drug Therapy — This is an important issue to address as there is a possibility that as a result of the surgery you may require continuing drug therapy. This is the time to address the side effects and possible complications of drug therapy as you may have to live with it for the rest of your life.

Implant Device Rejection — Ask about the possibility of rejection of your body of the implant device or the effect of scarring around the implant.

Procedure Risk — This is where you may want to ask what else can go wrong such as the nicking of an artery or puncturing an adjacent organ.

This type of risk may be referred to as iatrogenic (physician induced). It may be very difficult to know the physician's frequency of complications of this nature.

After you have a thorough discussion of the risks and complications you may want to consider all the facts and consider the possibility of a lifestyle change. Surgery may force a lifestyle change anyway. Or if you don't change your lifestyle, you may face surgery again.

Pain

* How much pain should I expect?

The typical physician response to this is "there may be some slight or minor discomfort," very few physicians can say "the pain will be excruciating and you will have difficulty walking for a few days." To get an answer to this question ask to rate the pain on a scale of 1 to 10 or ask what pain they have experienced and how it compares to what you should expect.

The patient can not determine if the surgery outcome is normal without some idea of the expected pain. If the patient is expecting "a minor discomfort" and the pain is worse, they may feel that surgery did not go well and wonder about its success.

Condition Recurrence Possibilities

* What are the chances of this condition reoccurring? And when?

Many times patients enter a treatment plan feeling they will be cured, but in five to ten years the condition reoccurs. It is important that you know if the treatment plan may only be temporary and might have to be performed again in the future. Many times a lifestyle change could eliminate the necessity for a repeat treatment plan.

Don't ask this question if you are pregnant or having your appendix removed. In the first case, the doctor has no idea of the chances of your becoming pregnant again, and, in the second, the patient knows the chances of growing a new appendix are extremely remote.

If the procedure is an angioplasty this is a valid question, since there is a 25 percent to 35 percent chance that the procedure will have to be repeated within six months.

Alternatives

*   What are my alternative treatment plans — physical therapy, medication, other surgeries?

A good lead-in to discussions of alternative treatments is to ask the question; "If this treatment (the one suggested) doesn't work, what's next?" This question also allows you to ask; "What is the probability of success of the suggested treatment?"

Of course both of these questions allow the patient to assess the reliability of the diagnosis and treatment in a quiet, assertive, inquisitive and non-threatening manner.

A recent study by the University of Minnesota illustrates different treatments can be suggested by different physician specialties. Two groups of doctors, surgical and nonsurgical specialists, were separated into two rooms. The two groups were presented with the same patient case study and were surveyed for their treatment plan suggestions. The surgical group recommended surgery and the nonsurgical group recommended nonsurgical treatment. The study clearly indicates that doctors may have a training and experience bias.

It is extremely beneficial if your doctor can supply written documentation concerning alternate treatment plans, scientific studies and articles supporting the indications for the alternate treatment plans, success rates and complication rates. Be sure and ask your doctor to provide documentation for and against your treatment plan.

You should not be afraid to ask for this pro and con data. Most of us review documentation when we are buying products such as TVs, electronic equipment and cars. We normally research these purchases thoroughly. We shouldn't be afraid to ask these same questions about treatment plans that can affect the future quality of our lives.

After reviewing the doctor supplied information, you should discuss why your doctor is recommending one course of treatment versus another. If your doctor does not supply scientific articles, you may search the medical databases. (See the chapter on computer retrieval of medical studies.)

How Much

*   How much will treatment cost?

Yes, here is that same question again. Now you need to ask how much the treatment will cost. It is much better to find out before treatment than after. You have no control of cost after treatment is provided. Your only recourse is to disagree or work out a payment schedule. If you ask before, at least you can make a value judgement.

It is much easier to discuss price with the doctor, than with the doctor's billing department. Billing departments have a notorious reputation for not negotiating. They expect you to pay the bill even though you bought the service without knowing the price.

When the price is given, ask which price? You should say that you expect the lowest billing rate, such as Medicare or managed care price.

If the physician won't give you those prices or they seem high, you may want to go "shopping" as you now have the diagnosis and suggested treatment with which you can shop. Also, be sure to get your medical records so you won't have to pay for an initial office visit with the next doctor.

Postpone Treatment

*   What will happen if I don't have the operation *now?*

*   How long can treatment be delayed? What would the result be?

Many times it is suggested that the treatment be scheduled immediately, particularly if it includes surgery. For many of us, this constitutes an emergency hospitalization. What will happen if you delay your decision one day, two weeks or forever? Many times surgery can be delayed while you obtain information about your condition and alternate treatment plans, or visit another doctor for a second opinion. If you wish to delay your treatment, you can ask that you own blood be used during surgery — this will delay treatment while you store your blood.

QUESTIONS IF DRUGS ARE PRESCRIBED

Ask for the spelling of the drug prescribed. This will allow you to use your medical library to get more information, and you can check that the pharmacy interpreted the doctor's handwriting correctly. Sometimes it is difficult to read the doctor's handwriting and this will assure a mistake hasn't been made.

****

<u>**CONCEPT AT WORK**</u>:

First Story — A patient returned for the follow-up visit after a doctor had prescribed medication for treatment of the daughter's right ear problem. The doctor noticed that the ear wasn't any better and asked the mother if she was applying the medication to the right ear. The mother said "right ear? I have been applying it to her bottom like the drug label says." The doctor looked at the label and it said "Apply drops to rear of child." The druggist had typed rear instead of r. ear and mom followed the instructions.

Second Story — A famous movie director suffered a mini breakdown caused by deep depression which was a side effect of a prescribed medication. When the medication was stopped he resumed normal activities but had lost a productive six months.

****

Drug Need

*   What will happen if I don't take drugs? Will my condition correct itself?

How Long?

*   How long will I be on medication? When will I start to fell better? What can I do to reduce the medication amount?

        This question is designed to lead into a discussion on lifestyle changes which could reduce your need for the drug. Many of the most frequently prescribed drugs can be reduced through lifestyle changes rather than a lifetime of maintenance drugs.

        Lifestyle changes have the additional benefit of improving your outlook and making you healthier without drug side effects.

When You Take Drug

*   Do I take it with or without food, before or after meals?
*   Should I avoid alcohol?
*   Will it react with any of my other medications?
*   What do I do if I forget to take the drug; take 2, take 1 at the normal time, or take 1 when I remember?

        All of these questions are important and may affect the effectiveness of your medications. It is best to write down these instructions as you most likely will forget if you don't. If you have a drug book in your medical library, most of these questions will be answered in the book and you won't have to always write down the instructions.

Drug Side Effects

*   What are the side effects of the drug? How will I feel?

It is extremely important that you thoroughly understand the side effects expected from the prescribed drug. Ask the physician to explain them to you, or better yet, ask for a copy of the pages from the doctor's *PDR (Physician's Desk Reference)*. If is very difficult for doctors to remember *all* the warnings for *all* the drugs. Besides, if you don't have a written copy you'll probably forget.

If you ask the pharmacist for a copy of the FDA warnings, it may result in receiving the warnings in print size most patients can't read.

This is an example of the type size used by one drug company to explain the dosages, side effects, warnings and cautions concerning who shouldn't take the drug. These written instructions are really important because studies show that 50 percent to 75 percent of patients forget what the doctor told them in the office. How can they expect a person over 40 to read this without a magnifying glass? There ought to be a law!

The above is this paragraph printed in a type size used by one drug company to explain the dosages, side effects, warnings and cautions concerning who shouldn't take the drug. These written instructions are really important because studies show that 50 percent to 75 percent of patients forget what the doctor told them in the office. How can they expect a person over 40 to read this without a magnifying glass? There ought to be a law!

It is important that you know the drug side effects, since you do not want to return to the physician with a symptom which in reality is only the side effect of the drug. Not only do you waste the physician's time, but you waste your own time and incur additional cost.

*   If you are taking more than three medications — why? It is suggested that you look at the *Physicians Desk Reference (PDR)* or your medical library for side effects and interactions.

Almost all drugs have a side effect. When you consume more than three drugs it becomes very difficult for the physician to determine whether he is treating your illness, a drug side effect or an interaction between two drugs.

The *PDR* is available in most libraries and presents side effect information in a clear way. After becoming aware of these side effects, you may be able to determine if you are suffering from a drug side effect or the symptom of an illness.

Drug Interaction

*   How will the drug interact with foods or alcohol? Should I avoid certain foods, drinks or alcohol?

Some drugs may be ineffective when taken with certain other substances or may cause a violent reaction, death or drowsiness that can lead to accidents.

Computer Analysis

* Will you perform a computer analysis of *all* the drugs I am taking to determine their interactions and reactions with each other?

It is possible for two beneficial drugs to react with each other and cause severe problems for the patient.

There are several computer programs now available to physician's offices that require only the names of the drugs to be entered. The software performs an analysis of the drug interactions, the reactions with other drugs or food and alcohol, and will also print the drug side effects on easy-to-read standard size computer paper. These programs cost only $400 to $1,000 per year to lease. If your doctor doesn't have one, ask him to get one. The cost per patient is very small and you can leave the office fully informed.

If your physician does not have a computer program of this type available, ask the same question of your pharmacy. It may even be better to ask the pharmacy, since it may have a record of all your medications and can easily run the computer analysis.

Drug Cost

* How much does the drug cost? Can I use something less expensive, such as a generic brand?

Free Samples

* Do you have any samples? May I try some?

Many times, doctors prescribe drugs in 30-day supplies which can be wasted if you have an unpleasant reaction or side effect. Why not start with a small supply to ensure that you have no allergies or side effects?

FDA Rating

* What is the FDA therapeutic *potential* rating?

    The FDA rates new drugs by the therapeutic gain/improvement over currently available drugs. This is their rating code:

> A = Important Therapeutic Gain
> B = Moderate Therapeutic Gain
> C = Little or No Therapeutic Gain

    A word of warning . . . The FDA also uses the A, B, C rating system to show therapeutic *equivalency* which is not the same as therapeutic *gain*. Equivalency means the drug has the same active ingredients and identical strength ("me too"). A brand new "break through" drug will be rated "A" for therapeutic *gain* and all the following "me too" drugs will be rated "B or C" for therapeutic *gain* because there is no therapeutic gain over the "break through" drug. Both the new drug and the "me too" drug will now have an "A" therapeutic *equivalency* rating because they are equivalent.

    Eighty-four percent of the 348 new drugs introduced between 1981 and 1988 received a "C" rating by the FDA (little or no therapeutic gain). (You can get the detailed August 1989 Staff Report of the U.S. Senate Special Committee on Aging entitled "Prescription Drug Prices: Are We Getting Our Money's Worth?" by contacting your U.S. Senator.) Since new drugs may cost up to ten times more than older drugs, it might be appropriate to ask your doctor for the FDA therapeutic *potential* rating. What patient wants to pay up to ten times more for a new "C" rated drug with little or no therapeutic gain? (If your doctor is not aware of the FDA rating, the drug manufacturer representative can provide this information.)

QUESTIONS IF TESTS ARE SUGGESTED

    Ask questions about the need for medical tests. Consider the results of three recent studies.

    The first study reported that approximately 25 percent of testing laboratories are partially or wholly owned by physicians.

    The second study reported that doctors who have x-ray equipment and ultrasound machines in their office order four times as many tests and charge more than doctors who don't have the equipment on-site.

    The third study reported that doctors who own labs and testing facilities order 14 percent more expensive lab tests and 82 percent more imaging tests than doctors who must refer patient out.

Companies who sell imaging equipment to physicians suggest that a leased $20,000 x-ray machine will generate an additional $200,000 in billings over a five year period. Physician ownership of lab and testing may have revenue considerations as well as patient convenience considerations. (At the current time there are no studies that show physician ownership of testing equipment improves patient outcomes.)

Test Necessary?

*   Is this test absolutely necessary *now?*

      You should thoroughly discuss testing with your doctor and determine if it is for your benefit or for the physician's (*i.e.,* future litigation protection).

What Results?

*   What results will you be looking for?
*   Will the test results determine or change your treatment plan?

      If the test results will not change the physician's treatment plan, you should question whether the test is necessary.

      Once you have determined the necessity for the test, discuss what normal test results are and how the physician will interpret the deviations.

*   Do the benefits of the test outweigh the risk or cost?
*   What are the dangers? Will there be any pain during the test procedure?

      This is an important question to ask if it is to be an "invasive" test. "Invasive" tests have a greater risk to the patient than "noninvasive" tests. A recent study at the University of California at San Francisco Medical School revealed that 14 percent of the patients who had an "invasive" test suffered at least one complication. Complications were infections, allergic reactions, unusual pain or death.

      If the patient has a 14 percent (1 out of 8) chance of a complication, the patient should feel that the test is necessary.

      Be sure you receive a copy of your test results. There have been occasions when test results revealed a serious, life-threatening illness and the patient was not notified due to some foul-up. Don't let this happen to you, besides you will want the results for your own medical records file.

Test Costs

*   How much does the test cost? Is there a less expensive, less risky first test?

     There is a great cost difference in imaging equipment. You should be sure that the increased cost will provide increased benefits.

Type of Equipment	Patient Cost	Cost to Purchase (Approximate/Average)
X-ray	$50 – $300	$80,000 ($28,000 to $150,000)
Ultrasound	$50 – $300	$80,000 ($13,000 to $250,000)
CT Scan (Computed tourography)	$300 – $900 Ea.	$1,100,000
MRI (Magnetic Resonance Imaging)	$800 – $1,500 Ea.	$2,200,000

     A quick calculation shows that 2,500 to 2,750 CT or MRI tests must be billed to pay for the purchase of the equipment, not including the labor and overhead. If tests are not run on the equipment, the equipment can not be paid for.

     As more and more physician testing equipment ownership occurs, cost will increase because fewer tests will be run on each piece of equipment. Look for the next cost and utilization escalation to occur in the area of medical tests.

Facility License

*   Is the facility licensed by the state or Medicare program?

     States normally license imaging facilities after checking the equipment, its calibration and the qualifications of the personnel. Some states estimate that 10 to 12 percent of the imaging facilities fail the licensing process due to miscalibrated or misaligned equipment and the use of unlicensed personnel.

Training Level

*   Who will read and interpret the test results?

Normally the state licenses the personnel based on their training and categories. Personnel who read and interpret the results are technicians, limited technicians, practical technicians, doctors and board certified doctors.

The newer type imaging equipment (CT scanners and MRIs) is so sophisticated and the reading of the results so complex that the technicians must be trained on that specific equipment.

Accuracy of Referred Lab

*   Why do you suggest this lab? What is the lab's accuracy rating? *You may be able to obtain a copy of state testing results from State Lab Licensing Department, if the lab does not respond to your request.*

It is common for test results to vary with different labs. This becomes extremely critical to you as a patient, since the results of the test may determine the course of treatment prescribed by the physician. If the lab has a poor accuracy testing rate (some states consider 75 percent a passing grade, a 25 percent inaccuracy rate), the physician may prescribe a treatment plan that is unnecessary or fail to provide a treatment plan when one may be necessary. You and your physician should therefore be aware of the lab's accuracy rating.

Most labs are tested using protocols and samples submitted by established testing programs of various organizations. The lab's ability to pass tests established by these organizations is one of the factors in the licensing process. These organizations have established lab proficiency programs:

Center for Disease Control (CDC)

College of American Pathology (CAP)

Institute of Toxicology

American Association of Bioanalyst (AAB)

American Academy of Family Physicians (AAFP–PT)

Medical Laboratory Evaluation Program (MLE)

American Society of Internal Medicine

American Society of Cytology

You may want to request the results of the last state or federal accuracy testing report from the lab. If the lab is hesitant to provide this information, ask your doctor to get it for you. If it is not provided, make that part of your decision.

Lab Personnel

* Who will test and interpret samples?

If you have lab work performed you want to know if the sample will be read and interpreted correctly.

Lab accuracy is a result of the equipment used, its calibration and the quality and training of the personnel testing the samples. Most state licensing agencies qualify the labs based on the accuracy of the testing equipment and the training qualifications of the personnel. The training and experience level of the personnel can range from an individual with very little training and education to a medical doctor.

Below are job titles commonly used in the medical testing industry and the associated training; normally the more training the more likely the interpretation will be correct:

Technician Trainee — An entry level position that requires a high school diploma or one year of college.

Technician — Requires at least two years as a technician trainee and two or less years of college work with courses in chemistry and biology.

Technologist — Normally three years of college or a degree in medical technology and some lab experience.

Toxicologist — Normally a Ph.D., with a degree in chemical or biological sciences.

Physician — A medical doctor, graduated from an accredited school.

SUMMARY

If you need surgery or medical treatment, your local library normally provides a good source of reference books or access to medical databases.

If you are having major surgery or treatment, a list of self-help groups may be available from hospitals, medical societies, or community health organizations. Self-help groups let you discuss your treatment plans, doctor selection and/or success rates *before* treatment and will be a source of help *after* treatment.

COST ESTIMATOR

The cost estimator form can be used to evaluate the cost of the recommended procedure and the alternative procedures. It is designed to highlight most of the areas from which costs may be incurred. It is particularly important that you get the correct cost when you get cost estimates. As an example, the retail cost may be quoted as $2,400. The physician, however, will accept $1,700 if paid by the insurance company and may accept less if he is a Preferred Provider "PPO" for the insurance company.

An easy way to get costs is to ask for a copy of a recent bill.

The healthcare industry is unique in it that price quotes tend to be on the high side and actual accepted payments are lower than quoted prices. Be sure that you and the provider are talking about the actual charges for which you will be responsible.

Reorder from: Med. Ed., Inc., P.O. Box 40696, Mesa, Arizona 85274

COST ESTIMATOR ™

Try to collect these costs before your treatment and review them with your primary doctor to see if he agrees (this may be the first time he sees the total cost of your treatment plan.)

As a general rule, your total hospital charges should be 6-10 times your room rate, so be sure you get an estimate of all hospital charges.

Medical Provider Name

DOCTORS						
Primary Care						
Specialist						
Surgeon						
Assistant Surgeon						
Radiologist						
Anesthesiologist						
Pathologist						
Follow-up visits						
DRUGS						
LAB WORK						
X-ray						
CAT Scan						
MRI						
Pathology						
Laboratory Test						
Other						
HOSPITAL						
Pre-admission test						
Required Tests (Before/After)						
Room rate						
Operating room (OR)						
Recovery room						
Intensive care room (ICU)						
Delivery room						
Birthing room						
"Stand-by" team						
HOSPITAL MISC. CHARGES						
Pharmacy						
Supplies (Medical/Surgery)						
Radiology						
Respiratory Therapy						
Physical Therapy						

COMPARISON OF
QUALITY AND SERVICE ISSUE FORM

Doctors	Doctor 1	Doctor 2
Provides Written Treatment Plan		
Provides Price Estimates		
Agrees to Waive Excess Fees		
Preferred Provider (PPO)		
Gives Copies of Medical Records		
ABMS Board Certified		
Designated Fellowship		
Performed Procedure _____ Times		
Provides Patient References		
Certified "Drug Free" Office		
Certified "AIDS Free" Office		
Member of Medical Society		
Uses PAs and NPs		
Provides Written Drug Warnings		
Has Drug Analysis Computer		
Accepts Medicare Assignments		
Number of Hospitals Admitted		
Provides Free Drug Samples		
Helps Qualify Labs and Hospitals		
Medical Board Record Checked		

Labs	Lab 1	Lab 2
State Licensed		
Medicare Licensed		
ACR Accredited		
Provides Accuracy Reports		
Tested By What Organizations		
Qualifications of Lab Personnel		
Provides Price Estimates		

NOTES

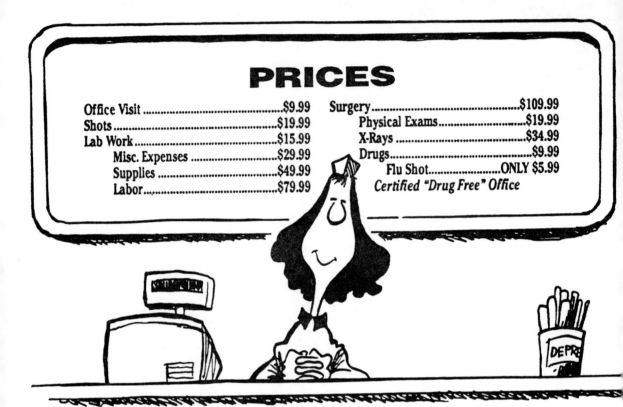

Wouldn't It Be Nice

CHAPTER 7

HOW MUCH? — A DIALOGUE

We would be remiss if we asked you to ask about medical prices and didn't coach you concerning some provider reactions to questions about costs.

The following dialogue offers some sample questions and responses that occur when the issue of price is discussed with healthcare providers.

Dialogue

Patient Q: How much?

Provider A: Pardon?

They can't believe you are asking about price. Nobody asks about price.

Patient Q: How much for (fill in blank)?

Provider A:

Alternative 1   Why do you care, your insurance will pay.

This will probably be the most common response and is really not as much a reflection of a non-caring attitude as it is an embarrassing question. Most healthcare providers don't know the cost of medical treatment. Some don't know their own cost and a majority have no idea about the costs of the hospitals and labs to which they are referring you.

99

Alternative 2 $2,500

> *You may now faint. Few doctors (and none voluntarily) give prices except for OB/GYNs for maternity care or cosmetic surgeons for surgery not covered by insurance. (Doesn't it seem strange that cosmetic surgeons know the cost of their services and other providers don't?)*

Patient A:

Best Answer   You mean you will accept my insurance payment as *full payment* and you won't try to collect the excess from me? Can I have that in writing?

> *This is a good patient response because of course you will have to pay something and you want to know before rather than after. This answer forces both the provider and the patient to acknowledge that treatment is not "free" and cost is a factor.*

Alternative 1   Because I care.

> *This answer won't get you anywhere, they won't believe you. Nobody cares about the cost of medical services.*

Alternative 2   Because I don't have insurance.

> *This will get their attention, maybe sympathy, maybe a lower price, and maybe less treatment, testing and drug expense.*

> *This is really a very effective way of getting only the necessary treatment and testing.*

> *This may be an appropriate response whenever you are having the initial doctor visits. Use your insurance only for very expensive items that you cannot afford such as hospital admittance.*

Alternative 3   Because I have a high deductible.

> *This may backfire as they may try to run up the bill to get you past your deductible so you won't ask the dumb question about price next time.*

> *You have to be careful here that they don't inflate the bill so much and allow you to waive your deductible as this is considered fraud and you would be participating in fraud.*

Alternative 4   Because I have only $xxx to spend.

> *This response shows you have placed some value on their services. It gives them a budget to work with and tells them you have limits. If they plan to exceed your budget they should tell you.*

Alternative 5   Do you know?

> *This is a good question to ask. If they say no, ask them to find out because (and then select one of the alternatives above). If they say yes, ask the question, how much?*

As you can see, getting prices from healthcare providers may be difficult because few patients ask and providers don't know other provider's prices. We have to start asking about prices, so that providers will start making price information available to patients.

There is an easy way to find out the cost of service, **simply ask for a copy of a previous patient's bill** (they can strike out the information which would identify the patient). This way you not only get the cost but you know the doctor has performed the procedure at least once. Asking for a copy of a previous bill should also work with other providers such as hospitals and labs.

DO NOT presume that "minor" outpatient surgery is inexpensive, below is an actual bill for a surgery of *less than one hour.*

Rooms		
Surgery Room (1 Hr. Min.) @	$756.26	
Recovery Room (1 Hr. Min.) @	200.80	
Total Rooms		**$ 957.06**
Miscellaneous		
Pharmacy	$ 615.60	
Surgical Supplies	1,107.64	
Lab/Test	111.10	
Anesthesia Supplies	233.70	
Total Hospital Outpatient		**$2,068.04**
Doctors		
Surgeon	$1,210.00	
Anesthetist	586.00	
Total Doctors		**$1,796.00**
Total Bill		**$4,821.10**

This bill illustrates how difficult it is for the healthcare consumer to comprehend the cost of medical treatment. If this patient asked the doctor about cost and was told the doctor's fee would be approximately $1,200, the patient would be shocked when the bill totaled $4,800. This patient was shocked not only at the size of the bill, but at their share of the cost, approximately $1,803 due to the deductible, co-insurance and excessive fees not covered by the insurance company. The patient was *really upset* about the $615.60 pharmacy bill, particularly when it was noted that the cost of one of the drugs was *four times* the price paid at a drug store.

How would you feel if you thought the bill would be approximately $1,200 and were presented a $4,800 bill for "minor" surgery?

This small bill illustrates the importance of asking about *all costs*.

The patient in this example was lucky, the providers were all PPO providers and excess charges were waived, saving almost $1,500.

NOTES

Your Best Friend

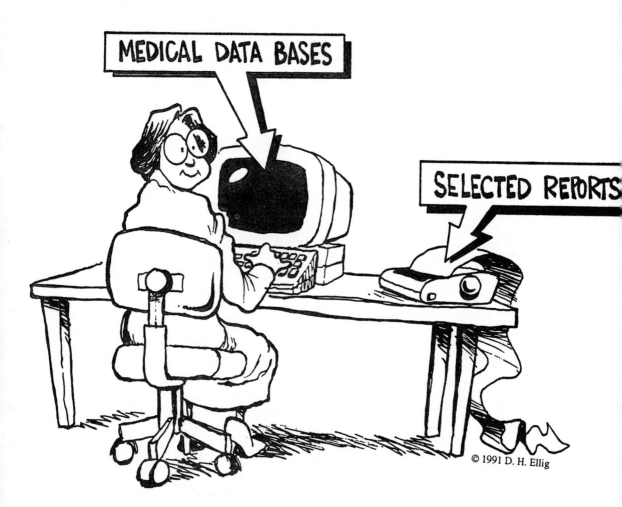

Marian the Librarian

CHAPTER 8

GETTING MORE INFORMATION

This may be the most important chapter in the book as the data revealed in this chapter will allow the patient to be truly informed and gather information that will allow the patient to ask intelligent questions about their treatment or condition. There is so much information available today at such a low cost that the patient no longer has to be feel intimidated as a result of their lack of knowledge.

The result of gathering this information is that the patient will feel more at ease with their treatment because they know the treatment is "the right thing to do," what their participation is in the treatment and that they participated in the decision.

Why This Chapter is Important

****

CONCEPT AT WORK:

First Story — Parent was told child needed surgery to correct a reoccurring ear problem. Parent went to a computer terminal and retrieved the most recently reported medical studies concerning the illness and the suggested surgery. Recent studies indicated that surgery procedure was only moderately successful and had later complications. Parent found that medical treatment with drugs could be as successful with none of the risk or later complications of surgery.

Discussion with doctor resulted in medical treatment with drugs rather than surgery.

Second Story — A patient entered the hospital for treatment of a heart condition. After five days of medical treatment with drugs the patient's condition had not improved and was considered for a heart transplant. A very high risk, complicated and expensive procedure.

A specialist was consulted and requested a computer search of the most recent medical studies. The search revealed that a medical treatment with different drugs may help.

The new treatment was successful and patient was discharged five days later. The computer search had found a treatment that cured the patient, and avoided the risk and cost of a heart transplant.

****

Why You Want the Studies

The important issue contained in the medical studies is *outcome probabilities*. It is easy for most of us to interpret probabilities.

A growing issue in good medical care is an informed patient. Unfortunately the current medical delivery system falls short of fully informing patients about their condition. Most of the time the doctor has all the information (or we think they have) and they simply make a decision about the "best" course of treatment for the patient, with very little patient input.

Research for this chapter revealed a sharp division in consumer medical information. Very little information is given to the patient and yet there is a wealth of patient information available. Most of the time the patient wants to know more, but is afraid to ask the doctor. Doctors normally discuss *why* you need the procedure and *how* it will be done, but little is mentioned about outcome probabilities, complications, or alternative treatments. The patient usually does not know where to get more information on his own. They can spend hours or days looking for help, yet all the information is available in medical studies.

These studies will reveal everything there is to know about your

condition
treatment plan
treatment plan success rates
latest treatments

— *but*

*were afraid to ask the doctor
and didn't know who to talk to or
where to go to get more information*

— and yet

*want to take an active part in their treatment and
want to make sure they are informed.*

Most medical studies will contain a high amount of medical jargon. It will be helpful if you have a consumer medical library which includes a medical dictionary and encyclopedia. The medical jargon should not be a deterrent to using these studies. Reading medical studies containing medical jargon will help us more intelligently discuss our condition with the physician. If these studies are read at home, at our leisure, there is much less intimidation than in the doctor's office.

You should not be afraid to discuss your condition or treatment with your doctor. Which thought would you rather have after medical treatment "I wish I would have asked" or "I am glad I asked"? Your doctor cannot be the "best and brightest" for *all* illnesses. The sources made available in this chapter provide an access to the "best and brightest" experts in the field. Their literature and research will help your doctor develop the best treatment plan for you with the latest data available. With so many public health care information data sources available there is no reason for a patient to be uninformed. An informed patient may help the physician select the best treatment plan for that individual patient from data provided by sources referenced in this chapter.

Consult
With the
World's Leading
Medical Authorities
$25 an hour
ALSO AVAILABLE:
House calls $25 an hour • At your office $25 an hour

What You Can Get

The ad for doctors at $25 per hour may appear too good to be true. How can it be possible to consult a doctor for only $25 per hour at your house or on the job, 24 hours a day.

These consultations will give you the results of many multimillion dollar scientific medical studies; all for only $25 per hour. All you will need is a computer or someone who can use a computer.

When you consult these medical studies you will know

what works
what doesn't work
what's new
what's being tested
where it's being tested
and
what are the outcome probabilities

The reason these doctors are so inexpensive is that you, or someone you hire, can retrieve the medical studies results via a computer terminal.

The medical delivery system is part of today's extensive computerization of facts and figures. Almost all articles published in the many medical journals and periodicals are retained for retrieval by computer. They are indexed by subject, so that articles published worldwide can be referenced and retrieved from databases.

The availability of large amounts of reference materials and research studies can help you intelligently discuss alternatives with your physicians. These articles are an excellent source for the physician and the patient to obtain information about the latest treatment plans, treatment centers and information about the success of the treatment plans.

As an example of the applicability of computer retrieval of medical studies, we requested information concerning natural childbirth after a previous delivery via cesarian. The computer inquiry retrieved 42 articles referencing numerous studies concerning the advisability, parameters and possibilities of natural birth after cesarian. The cost was $38.00. (It was interesting to note that some of the studies indicated that the cesarian surgical procedure was the most frequently performed surgical procedure in the United States. Even more interesting is the fact that cesarians can be performed on only half of the population.)

How to Access Studies

There are several ways to gain access to this large body of previously published studies. There are four primary methods and sources for retrieving these medical studies:

> at the library
> in your home
> hire someone
> at your employer

Library — Help is available at your local library, which is a rich source of medical data. If the library has computer access to medical studies, the patient has hit the "gold mine." This wealth of information is available to everyone.

Of course the library will be the least expensive as it is free. Many libraries now provide computer access to many reference sources. One of these reference sources is medical information. Most libraries will use either the *Info-Trac Health* or the *Health Resource System.* Both of these systems are extremely easy to use and a librarian will show you how to use the computer. Any studies of interest may be printed by the library's computer printers. You need only push the print button.

At Home — If you have a home computer with a modem you may directly access all of the sources for medical studies at the end of this chapter. The cost of a search is very minimal. The largest and most complete database (6.5 million articles), MEDLINE, charges only $25 per hour. Most searches require only five to ten minutes if you use a search help program. This means that for $5 to $10 you can receive 20 to 50 medical study abstracts that cost millions of dollars to research.

Search help programs are beneficial as they are designed to help the novice develop a search argument while off line. You are charged only for search time, not for the time while you construct the search argument (tells the computer which type of study you want).

The number and extent of data sources containing medical literature is extensive and separate programs have been developed to help analysts search for information.

Some of the search help programs are:

GRATEFUL MED — This particular program makes it easy to search MEDLINE and was developed by the National Library of Medicine. It helps the user develop search parameters. When the user is satisfied with the parameters, Grateful Med will enter the MEDLINE system, retrieve the data, down load the data and sign off. This keeps user search cost low.

The search programs can be purchased for $29.95 plus $3.00 in shipping from the National Technical Information Service, 5285 Port Royal Road, Springfield, VA 22161.

PAPER CHASE — This is an on-line search help service available by subscription. It was developed by librarians at Beth Israel Hospital in Boston.

If you want the full text of an article you may order it using Paper Chase. Paper Chase is also available through CompuServe. Information is available from Beth Israel Hospital, 333 Brookline Ave., Boston, MA 02215, (617) 735-2253.

EASYNET — This system was developed to provide easy access to the hundreds of databases on BRS, DIALOG and other vendors. It is also available through CompuServe as IQUEST or you may contract directly with Easynet simply by having your computer call 800-EASYNET and provide a charge card number.

For more information contact Telebase Systems, 763 W. Lancaster Ave., Bryn Mawr, PA 19010, (800) 841-9553 or (215) 526-2800.

Hire Someone — The third alternative is to hire someone to search for the study topics you want. Some people may not have access to libraries with computers or have home computers. They may hire a search analyst firm to retrieve the most recent medical studies. The prices charged by these firms are normally quite reasonable and compared to the cost of medical treatment, very reasonable. There are firms called database vendors who allow users to access medical studies for a fee.

Simply call a database vendor for a list of their users in your area. Then call one, determine rates and procedures, and within a day or two you will receive the results of the computer retrieval of medical studies concerning your treatment or condition.

Database Vendors List

BRS Information Technologies
1200 Route 7
Latham, NY 12110
(800) 345-4BRS

BRS/Saunders Colleague
555 East Lancaster Avenue
St. Davids, PA 19087
(215) 254-0236

CompuServe Information Service
5000 Arlington Centre Blvd.
P.O. Box 20212
Columbus, OH 43220
(800) 848-8199
in Ohio (614) 457-0802

DIALOG Information Services
Marketing Department
3460 Hillview Avenue
Palo Alto, CA 94304
(800) 334-2564

EasyNet
Telebase Systems
763 W. Lancaster Avenue
Bryn Mawr, PA 19010
(800) 841-9553
(215) 526-2800

MEDIS
Mead Data Central
19393 Springboro Pike
P.O. Box 933
Dayton, OH 45401
(513) 865-6800

National Library of Medicine
MEDLARS Management Section
Building 38, Room 4N42
18600 Rockville Pike
Bethesda, MD 20894
(800) 638-8480
(301) 496-6193

Health Reference Center and
Info-Trac Health
Information Access Company
362 Lakeside Drive
Foster City, CA 94404
(800) 441-1165 (U.S.A.)
(800) 227-8431 (Canada)

Employers/Doctors — It is possible that some employers may have one of the medical databases available, or an individual who can access the MEDLINE database, or have a contract with a search analyst firm. Your doctor also has access to the MEDLINE database, either at his office, or through the hospital. At the current time, doctors and hospitals are the greatest users of the MEDLINE computer retrieval system. You can ask your doctor to retrieve the most recent studies, however, the doctor may resist as it will take more time and the studies may conflict with his recommendations. Some patients may also feel uncomfortable asking a doctor to retrieve studies. In either case you will have to use one of the three other retrieval methods.

Data Available

We are providing a list of data sources, the type of data and the database vendors. We provide this information so that you can see the extent of information available to you, as an example, if you have a particular need for specific information about a rare disease, it can be retrieved through the rare disease database.

The National Health Information Center publishes a free pamphlet "On-Line Health Information" which lists more databases than we have here. Ask for the health finder when you write or call for information:

National Health Information Center
P.O. Box 1133
Washington, DC 20013
(301) 565-4167 in MD or (800) 336-4797

MEDICAL DATABASES

> **Warning** — This information is the latest available at the time this book was printed. Because of the rapid changing technology some of the data contained herein may change, i.e., improved access, more data available, more full text. It is suggested that you confirm the information shown with database vendors or your search analyst.

AGELINE
    Citations — Yes Abstracts — Yes Full Text — No
Data Available: Database contains references applicable for the middle age and aging populations. Describes federally funded research projects, plus references to economics, family relationships, demographic trends and health care.
    Size: 28,000 records
    Sources: American Association of Retired Persons
    Vendors: BRS, DIALOG

AIDSLIN
    Citations — Yes Abstracts — Yes Full Text — No
Data Available: The database references issues on the clinical and research aspects of AIDS and health policy issues.
    Size: 24,000 records
    Sources: U.S. National Library of Medicine
    Vendors: DIALOG, National Library of Medicine

BIOSIS PREVIEWS
Citations — Yes Abstracts — Yes Full Text — No
Data Available: Contains citations on all aspects of biosciences and medical research on a worldwide basis.
    Size: 6,000,000 records
    Sources: Biosis
    Vendors: BRS, DIALOG

CANCERLIT
Citations — Yes Abstracts — Yes Full Text — Yes
Data Available: Contains references to all cancer related articles on a worldwide basis to include experimental and clinical cancer therapy.
    Size: 700,000 records
    Sources: U.S. National Library of Medicine
    Vendors: BRS, DIALOG, National Library of Medicine

CLINPROT
Citations — Yes Abstracts — Yes Full Text — Yes
Data Available: Provides summary of clinical investigations of new cancer therapies. Designed primarily for cancer researchers who are engaged in the development and testing of cancer treatment programs.
    Size: 7,000 protocols
    Sources: NIH, National Cancer Institute
    Vendors: National Library of Medicine

CHILD ABUSE AND NEGLECT
Citations — Yes Abstracts — Yes Full Text — Yes
Data Available: Database has five subfiles, research project descriptions, program descriptions, availability of audio visual materials, legal references and articles.
    Size: 17,000 records
    Sources: National Center on Child Abuse and Neglect, U.S. Dept. of Health
                   and Human Services
    Vendors: DIALOG

CLINICAL ABSTRACTS
Citations — Yes Abstracts — Yes Full Text — No
Data Available: Data provided is oriented to the practicing physicians and major subject areas are pediatrics, family practice, internal medicine, general surgery and cardiovascular surgery.
    Size: 15,000 records
    Sources: Medical Information Systems, Reference and Index Services Inc.
    Vendors: DIALOG

COMBINED HEALTH INFORMATION DATABASE (CHID)
Citations — Yes Abstracts — Yes Full Text — Yes
Data Available: A combined database providing information on digestive diseases, arthritis and diabetes. Also provides health information and educational resources and provides information on organizations, publications, and programs.
A good source for disease-oriented information.
Size: N/A
Sources: Information is supplied by at least seven national disease-oriented organizations including Center for Disease Control, National Diabetes Information, National Digestive Diseases
Vendors: BRS

COMPREHENSIVE CORE MEDICAL LIBRARY
Citations — Yes Abstracts — Yes Full Text — Yes
Data Available: This is a full text database of major medical periodicals, textbooks and journals such as the *Lancet, Grays Anatomy,* and *Current Therapy.*
Size: N/A
Sources: W.B. Saunders
Vendors: BRS, BRS/Saunders College

DIRLIN
Citations — Yes Abstracts — Yes Full Text — Yes
Data Available: An excellent reference source for health organizations that provide help and information in many health care fields.
Size: N/A
Sources: Library of Congress and National Health Information Center
Vendors: National Library of Medicine, BRS, DIALOG

EMBASE
(formerly EXECRPTA MEDICA)
Citations — Yes Abstracts — Yes Full Text — No
Data Available: A source for searching medical literature produced on a worldwide basis. Provides references to articles in over 4,000 journals.
Size: 4,000,000 records
Sources: Execrpta Medica
Vendors: BRS, BRS/Saunders, Colleague DIALOG

EXPERTNET
Citations — Yes Abstracts — Yes Full Text — Yes
Data Available: This database contains a biographical profile of over a thousand medical experts willing to perform medicolegal consultation.
They represent virtually all medical specialists. Physician profiles are provided, such as medical specialty, training and board certification.

While this database is used primarily for legal search and expert witness research assistance it may provide a source for experts in particular fields.
Size: 1,274
Sources: Expertnet
Vendors: DIALOG

F-D-C REPORTS
Citations — Yes Abstracts — Yes Full Text — Yes
Data Available: Database includes the full text of FDA recalls and court actions plus the pink sheet®, gray sheet® and rose sheet®. This database is a reference source for most FDA activities and publications.
Size: 24,000 records
Sources: FDC Reports, Inc.
Vendors: DIALOG

HEALTH DEVICES ALERTS
Citations — Yes Abstracts — Yes Full Text — Yes
Data Available: Data includes reports of problems with implanted medical devices and related accessories, as well as diagnostic and therapeutic medical equipment. Covers most medical equipment and devices.
Size: 120,000 records
Sources: ECRI
Vendors: DIALOG

HEALTH LAWYER
Citations — Yes Abstracts — Yes Full Text — Yes
Data Available: Covers issues in health care law including case digests and references to journals, newsletters, etc.
Size: N/A
Sources: American Hospital Association, Office of Legal Communication
Vendors: BRS

HEALTH PERIODICALS DATABASE
Citations — Yes Abstracts — Yes Full Text — Yes
Data Available: Database contains a broad range of health subjects and issues collected from national publications. The Health Reference Database is an excellent consumer oriented database. National publication articles have been summarized and rewritten without the complex medical jargon (**may be available** at your library).
Size: 164,000 records
Sources: Information Access Company
Vendors: DIALOG

HEALTH REFERENCE CENTER (See Health Periodicals Database)

MEDLINE
Citations — Yes Abstracts — Yes Full Text — Yes
Data Available: This is the "granddaddy" of all medical information databases. This database covers virtually every subject in the broad field of medicine and indexes articles from journals throughout the world.
Size: 6,500,000 records
Sources: U.S. National Library of Medicine
Vendors: Almost all

MENTAL HEALTH ABSTRACTS
Citations — Yes Abstracts — Yes Full Text — Some
Data Available: Contains information on the treatment of mental health gathered from worldwide journals.
This is the mental health counterpart to MEDLINE.
Size: 500,000 records
Sources: National Clearing House for Mental Health Information
Vendors: Nearly all

NTIS
Citations — Yes Abstracts — Yes Full Text — No
Data Available: Database provides information on reports available from government agencies as provided through government sponsored research development and engineering programs.
Size: 1,400,000 records
Sources: National Technical Information Services, U.S. Department of Commerce
Vendors: BRS, DIALOG

PDQ (Physician Data Query)
Citations — Yes Abstracts — Yes Full Text — Yes
Data Available: This database was designed for direct use by physicians but is also available to the public. Data is cancer related and has four subfiles: 1) summaries of major tumor types including treatment options; 2) directory of cancer specialists; 3) a directory of organizations associated with cancer treatment; and 4) cancer treatment methods approved by the National Cancer Institute.
Size: N/A
Sources: National Cancer Institute, National Institutes of Health
Vendors: National Library of Medicine, BRS/Saunders Colleague, MEDIS

PsycINFO
(Formerly Psychological Abstracts)
　　Citations — Yes　Abstracts — Yes　Full Text — No
Data Available: A database of articles on psychology and the behavioral health sciences.
　　Size:　　　700,000 records
　　Sources:　American Psychological Association
　　Vendors:　BRS, DIALOG

RARE DISEASE DATABASE
　　Citations — Yes　Abstracts — Yes　Full Text — Yes
Data Available: Provides information and indications of approximately 200 rare diseases. Includes general description, symptoms, therapy and references.
　　Size:
　　Sources:　National Organization for Rare Diseases
　　Vendors:　CompuServe

Drug Databases

CONSUMER DRUG INFORMATION FULL TEXT
　　Citations — Yes　Abstracts — Yes　Full Text — Yes
Data Available: Full text description of drugs telling how they work, possible side effects, precautions and instructions for taking them.
　　There is also a professional version of this called "Drug Information Full Text."
　　Size:　　　N/A
　　Sources:　American Society of Hospital Pharmacists
　　Vendors:　BRS, DIALOG

DRUGINFO
　　Citations — Yes　Abstracts — Yes　Full Text — No
Data Available: A drug/alcohol use and abuse database, providing information about psychological aspects of therapy and treatments.
　　Size:　　　N/A
　　Sources:　Drug Information Services, College of Pharmacy, University of
　　　　　　　Minnesota
　　Vendors:　BRS

SEDBAS
 Citations — Yes Abstracts — Yes Full Text — Yes
Data Available: Database documents every reported drug with side effects as reported in literature. Each year approximately 9,000 articles are written on adverse drug reactions. These articles are then reviewed and compressed for the key issues.
 Database covers drug reactions, interactions, special risks and toxicity.
 Size: 45,000 records
 Sources: Elsevier Science Publishers
 Vendors: DIALOG

DE HAEN'S DRUG DATA
 Citations — Yes Abstracts — Yes Full Text — Yes
Data Available: Database provides information about adverse drug reactions, clinical studies, drug interactions and research study results of new drugs.
 Size: 89,000 records
 Sources: Paul de Haen International Inc.
 Vendors: DIALOG

Rehab Databases

ABELDATA
 Citations — Yes Abstracts — No   Full Text — No
Data Available: This is a source for information on rehabilitation products and technical aids for disabled persons. Provides a list of manufacturers, distributors and costs.
 Size: N/A
 Sources: National Rehabilitation Information Center
 Vendors: BRS

REHABDATA (NARIC)
 Citations — Yes Abstracts — Yes Full Text —
Data Available: Provides sources for articles on physically and mentally disabled conditions.
 Size: 22,000
 Sources: National Rehabilitation Information Center
 Vendors: BRS

How to Evaluate Credibility of Study

Use of these databases will provide a number of studies. It is important that you understand how to evaluate the credibility of the studies using the following factors. If there are a number of studies the preponderance of the study results should be considered.

1.   Size of study. The larger the study the better.

2.   Length of study. The longer the study and follow-up, the better.

3.   Use of control group. The better studies have three groups; the control group, the treatment group and the group having a "placebo" treatment.

4.   A double-blind study. This type of study requires that both the researchers and the participants not know who is receiving the treatment or the placebo.

5.   Random assignment of study participants. This is to ensure impartial selectivity of the participants.

6.   Age and sex of study group. Compare the study group to ensure that the participants being studied are comparable to your age and sex, as treatment results can vary by age, sex and ethnic group.

7.   Funding source of study. If you can find this out you can make your own determination as to any possible study bias.

8.   Number of studies. Generally there are many studies on a given treatment plan. The more studies, the better.

9.   Consistency of findings. There should be a consistency of findings.

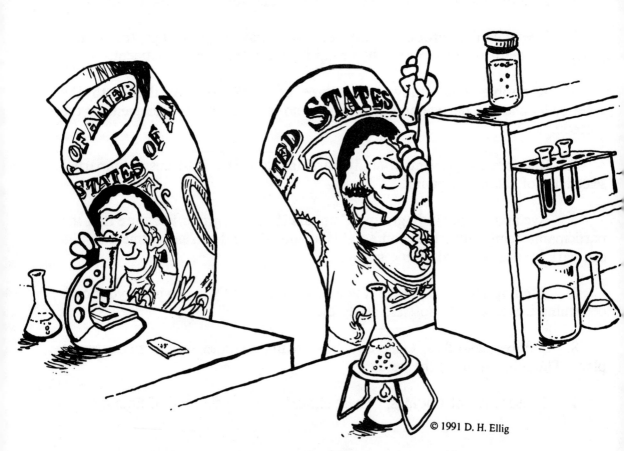

© 1991 D. H. Ellig

"U.S. Tax Dollars at Work"

CHAPTER 9

DISEASE RESEARCH RESOURCES

The United States government does an absolutely fantastic job funding medical research. Most medical research is done through the National Institute of Health. This is an extremely large organization with many, many branches specializing and researching many diseases.

The sources listed below include research sources which you may contact for either written documentation, referral to the latest treatment programs or research centers. Some national disease specific organizations are also provided. These sources provide an ideal starting point from which to gather the most current information about your illness, condition, disease or problem. **Most provided at no charge!**

Most of these referrals are federally funded. If a toll-free number is provided, expect a frequent busy signal. Keep trying. It will be worth it.

The NIH (National Institutes of Health) Publications List (#8907) is a free catalog, listing the addresses, phone numbers and publications available from each of the Institutes. It is available at

PUBLICATIONS FROM ALL NIH INSTITUTES
Public Information Division
National Institute of Health, Room 305
Bethesda, MD 20892
(301) 496-4143

The following are some of the Disease Research Referral sources listed in the above publication, plus some additional sources:

AGING

National Institute on Aging
NIH, Federal Building Room 6C12
Bethesda, MD 20892
(301) 496-1752

Self-Help for the Elderly
640 Pine Street
San Francisco, CA 94108
(415) 982-9172

American Association for Retired Persons
National Gerontology Resource Center
1909 K Street N.W.
Washington, DC 20049
(202) 728-4880

AIDS

Prevention
National AIDS Information
Clearinghouse
P.O. Box 6003
Rockville, MD 20850
(301) 762-5111
(800) 458-5231

Research Worldwide
National Institute of Allergy and
Infectious Diseases
NIH, Bldg. 31, Room 7A32
9000 Rockville Pike
Bethesda, MD 20892
(301) 496-5717

ALLERGIES AND INFECTIOUS DISEASES

National Institute of Allergy and
Infectious Diseases
NIH, Bldg. 31, Room 7A32
9000 Rockville Pike
Bethesda, MD 20892
(301) 496-5717

ALZHEIMERS

NIH
Adear Center
P.O. Box 8250
Silver Spring, MD 20907

ANOREXIA NERVOSA AND BULIMIA

National Institute of Child Health and
Human Development
NIH, Building 31, Room 2A-32
Bethesda, MD 20892
(301) 496-5133

APNEA AND SIDS

National Sudden Infant Death Syndrome
Clearinghouse
8201 Greensboro Drive, Suite 600
McLean, VA 22102
(202) 625-8410

ARTHRITIS

National Arthritis, Musculoskeletal &
Skin Disease Information Clearinghouse
P.O. Box 9782
Arlington, VA 22209
(703) 558-4999

Arthritis Foundation
1314 Spring Street N.W.
Atlanta, GA 30309
1-800-283-7800

ASTHMA AND RESPIRATORY DISORDERS

National Institute of Allergy and
Infectious Diseases
NIH, Bldg. 31, Room 7A32
9000 Rockville Pike
Bethesda, MD 20892
(301) 496-5717

BLINDNESS AND VISION PROBLEMS
National Eye Institute
Building 31, Room 6A32
9000 Rockville Pike
Bethesda, MD 20892
(301) 496-5248

BONE AND ORTHOPEDICS
Musculoskeletal Diseases Program
National Institute of Arthritis and
Musculoskeletal and Skin Diseases
Westwood Building, Room 407
Bethesda, MD 20205
(301) 496-4236

BOWEL DISEASE AND SYNDROME
National Digestive Diseases Information
Clearinghouse
Box NDDIC
Bethesda, MD 20892
(301) 468-6344

BRAIN TUMORS
National Institute of Neurological
Disorders and Stroke
NIH, Bldg. 31, 8A06
9000 Rockville Pike
Bethesda, MD 20892
(301) 496-4697

CANCER
Information
  Office of Cancer Communications
  National Cancer Institute
  Building 31, Room 10A18
  9000 Rockville Pike
  Bethesda, MD 20892
  (301) 496-5583

Detection and Diagnostic Imaging
  Diagnostic Imaging Research
  Program
  National Cancer Institute
  Executive Plaza North, Room 800
  6130 Executive Board
  Rockville, MD 20892
  (301) 496-9531

Chemotherapy, Radiation, Surgery
  Office of Clinical Center
  Communications
  Warren G. Magnuson Clinical Center
  NIH, Building 10, Room 5C-305
  9000 Rockville Pike
  Bethesda, MD 20892
  (301) 496-2563

CARDIOVASCULAR DISEASES
National Heart, Lung and Blood Institute
NIH, Building 31, Room 42-21
9000 Rockville Pike
Bethesda, MD 20892
(301) 496-4236

CEREBRAL PALSY
National Institute of Neurological
Disorders and Stroke
NIH, Bldg. 31, Room 8A06
9000 Rockville Pike
Bethesda, MD 20892
(301) 496-4697

CROHN'S DISEASE
National Digestive Diseases Information
Box NDDIC
Bethesda, MD 20892
(301) 468-6344

DIABETES
Information
  National Diabetes Information
  Clearinghouse
  Box NDIC
  Bethesda, MD 20892
  (301) 468-2162

Control Programs
  Division of Diabetes Translation
  Office of Chronic Disease
  Prevention and Health Promotion
  CDC, 1600 Clifton Rd., E08
  Atlanta, GA 30333
  (404) 639-1848

DIGESTIVE DISEASES
National Digestive Diseases Information
Box NDDIC
Bethesda, MD 20892
(301) 468-6344

DOWN'S SYNDROME
National Institute of Child Health and
Human Development
NIH, Building 31, Room 2A32
9000 Rockville Pike
Bethesda, MD 20892
(301) 496-5133

EYE AND VISION
NIH
Building 31, Room 6A32
9000 Rockville Pike
Bethesda, MD 20892
(301) 496-5248

Eye Research Experiments
National Eye Institute
NIH, Bldg. 31, Room 6A-32
9000 Rockville Pike
Bethesda, MD 20892
(301) 492-5248

HEAD INJURY
Musculoskeletal Diseases Program
National Inst. of Arthritis and
Musculoskeletal and Skin Diseases
Westwood Building, Room 407
Bethesda, MD 20205
(301) 496-5717

HEADACHES
American Council for Headache
Education
875 Kings Highway, Suite 200
West Deptford, NJ 08096
1-800-225-ACHE

HEART
Transplants
National Heart, Lung and Blood
Institute
NIH, Bldg. 31, Room 5A-52
9000 Rockville Pike
Bethesda, MD 20892
(301) 496-4236

Heart, Lung and Blood
National Heart, Lung and Blood
Institute
Building 31, Room 4A-21
9000 Rockville Pike
Bethesda, MD 20892
(301) 496-4236

HEMOPHILIA
National Hemophiliac Foundation
19 W. 34th Street, Suite 1204
New York, NY 10011
(212) 563-0211

HUNTINGTON'S DISEASE
Department of Medical Genetics
Indiana University Medical School
Medical Research Building
975 W. Walnut St.
Indianapolis, IN 46202
(317) 274-2245

INFERTILITY
Office of Consumer Affairs
Food and Drug Administration
Public Inquiries
5600 Fishers Lane (HFE-88)
Rockville, MD 20857
(301) 443-3170

KIDNEY AND UROLOGICAL DISEASES
National Kidney & Urological Diseases
Info. Clearinghouse
Box NKUDIC
Bethesda, MD 20892
(301) 468-6345

KIDNEY AND UROLOGICAL DISEASES — Continued

Stones and Transplants
National Institute of Diabetes
Digestive and Kidney Diseases
NIH, Building 31, Room 9A-04
9000 Rockville Pike
Bethesda, MD 20892
(301) 496-3583

LUNG TRANSPLANTS

National Heart, Lung and Blood Institute
NIH, Bldg. 31, Room 5A-52
9000 Rockville Pike
Bethesda, MD 20892
(301) 496-4236

MENTAL HEALTH

National Institute of Mental Health
Alcohol, Drug Abuse and Mental Health
Administration
5600 Fishers Lane, Room 15C05
Rockville, MD 20857
(301) 443-4515

Anger and Aggression
National Institute of Mental Health
Public Inquiries Branch
Parklawn Building
5600 Fishers Lane Room 15C-05
Rockville, MD 20857
(301) 443-4513

Depression
National Institute of Mental Health
Alcohol, Drug Abuse and Mental
Health Administration
5600 Fishers Lane, Room 15C05
Rockville, MD 20857
(301) 443-4515

Schizophrenia Research
Schizophrenia Research Branch
Division of Clinical Research
National Institute of Mental Health
Parklawn Building, Room 10C-16
5600 Fishers Lane
Rockville, MD 20857
(301) 443-4707

MENTAL RETARDATION RESEARCH

Mental Retardation Research Centers
National Institute of Child Health and
Human Development
Executive Plaza North, Room 631
6130 Executive Blvd.
Bethesda, MD 20897
(301) 496-1383

MUSCULOSKELETAL DISEASES

National Institute for Arthritis and
Musculoskeletal and Skin Diseases
NIH, Bldg. 31, Room 4C05
9000 Rockville Pike
Bethesda, MD 20892
(301) 496-8188

PREGNANCY AND ULTRASOUND TESTING

National Institute of Child Health and
Human Development
Office of Research Reporting
Building 31, Room 2A-32
9000 Rockville Pike
Bethesda, MD 20892
(301) 496-5133

PROSTATE

National Kidney & Urologic Diseases
Information
Box NKUDIC
9000 Rockville Pike
Bethesda, MD 20892
(301) 468-6345

RHEUMATIC DISEASE

National Institute of Arthritis and
Musculoskeletal Diseases
NIH, Building 31, Room 9A-04
Bethesda, MD 20892
(301) 496-5717

SICKLE CELL
National Sickle Cell Disease Program
7550 Wisconsin Ave., Room 504
Bethesda, MD 20892
(301) 496-6931

SPEECH AND LANGUAGE DISORDERS
National Institute on Deafness and
Other Communicative Disorders
NIH, Building 31, Room 1B62
9000 Rockville Pike
Bethesda, MD 20892
(301) 496-7243

SPINA BIFIDA
National Institute of Neurological
Disorders and Stroke
NIH, Bldg. 31, Room 8A06
9000 Rockville Pike
Bethesda, MD 20892
(301) 496-4697

SPINAL CORD INJURY
National Institute of Neurological
Disorders and Stroke
NIH, Bldg. 31, Room 8A06
9000 Rockville Pike
Bethesda, MD 20892
(301) 496-4697

STROKE AND BRAIN DISORDERS
National Institute of Neurological
Disorders and Stroke
NIH, Building 31, Room 8A06
9000 Rockville Pike
Bethesda, MD 20892
(301) 496-4697

SUDDEN INFANT DEATH SYNDROME (SIDS)
National Sudden Infant Death Syndrome
Clearinghouse
8201 Greensboro Dr., Suite 600
McLean, VA 22102
(703) 821-8955

ULCERS: GASTRIC AND DUODENAL
National Digestive Diseases Information
Box NDDIC
Bethesda, MD 20892
(301) 468-6344

MISCELLANEOUS CONTACTS
Below are additional organizations that
may be helpful:

American Medical Association
535 N. Dearborn Street
Chicago, IL 60610
(312) 645-5000

Centers for Disease Control
1600 Clifton Road, N.E.
Atlanta, GA 30333
(404) 329-3311

Veteran's Administration
Washington, DC 20420

NOTES

Don't Go It Alone

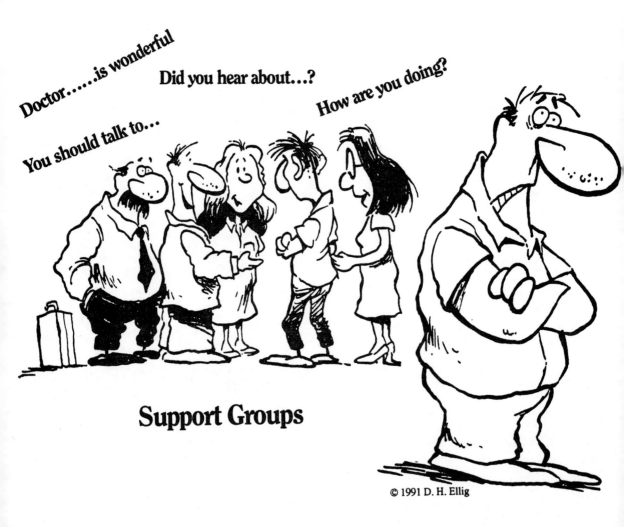

CHAPTER 10

DON'T GO IT ALONE

Support groups and illness specific foundations and associations are an important source of reference material provided by people and organizations who have gained a body of knowledge concerning specific conditions. These groups and organizations can be used to discuss:

doctors	success rates
hospitals	patient and family experiences
alternate treatment plans	

They can play a vital role in coping with illnesses by sharing emotional experiences. The groups also provide a wealth of consumer information and experience about the healthcare industry.

Why This Chapter is Important

****

CONCEPT AT WORK:

First Story — A patient with Parkinson's Disease who belonged to a Parkinson's Disease support group stated that he received ten times more information from the group than he did from his physician (even though the physician was a leading Parkinson's Disease expert). He indicated that this may be due to the fact that he spends more time and has a more intimate relationship with his support group than he does with the physician.

Second Story — An individual's parent suffered a sudden unexpected debilitating condition while on an out-of-town trip. The individual called a local community referral service. The individual received information about the condition, providers, treatments and sources for rehabilitation.

****

Toll-free support group numbers are listed for your reference as a starting point for self-education. This is only a partial list and is offered as an example of groups available to help you with specific problems. A more complete list is available free of charge from:

Hotlines/TW
NLM Information Office
8600 Rockville Pike
Bethesda, MD 20894

Be sure to also check local listings and ask hospitals and community health programs for their lists or referrals. Most communities and all states have organizations that maintain a list of local self-help groups and community help resources. To find a community help program call the United Way at (703) 836-7100 or The Alliance of Information and Referral Systems at (815) 744-6922.

All telephone numbers shown were current at the date of publication, however, may change. You may call 1-800-555-1212 for help if numbers have changed.

AIDS
National AIDS Hot Line
(800) 342-AIDS

ALCOHOL
Alcohol Rehab for the Elderly
(800) 354-7089
Al-Anon Family Group Headquarters
(800) 344-2666
Al-Anon/Al-Ateen
(800) 356-9996
National Council on Alcoholism
(800) NCA-CALL

ALCOHOL — Continued
See Local Listing
AA (Alcoholics Anonymous)
Al-Anon
Al-Ateen
Women for Sobriety

ALZHEIMER'S DISEASE
Alzheimer's Disease Assoc.
(800) 621-0379

ARTHRITIS
Arthritis Foundation
(800) 283-7800

ASTHMA
National Asthma Center
(800) 222-5864

BLINDNESS — See **SIGHT**

BULEMIA, ANOREXIA
Bulemia Anorexia Self-Help (B.A.S.H.)
(800) BASH-STL

CANCER
American Cancer Society
(800) 227-2345
Cancer Information Service
(800) 4-CANCER
Y-Me Breast Cancer Support Program
(800) 221-2141

CEREBRAL PALSY
United Cerebral Palsy Assoc.
(800) USA-1UCP

CHILD ABUSE
Child Abuse Hot Line
(800) 422-4453
National Hot Line for Missing and
Exploited Children
(800) 843-5678
Parents Anonymous
(800) 421-0353

CHILDREN
Institute of Logopedics
(800) 835-1043
National Center for Youth with
Disabilities (NCYD)
(800) 333-NCYD
National Information Center for
Children and Youth with Handicaps
(800) 999-5599
Tough Love
(800) 333-1069

CLEFT PALATE
Cleft Palate Foundation
(800) 242-5338

CYSTIC FIBROSIS
Cystic Fibrosis Foundation
(800) FIGHT-CF

DEAFNESS — See **HEARING**

DIABETES
American Diabetes Assoc.
(800) 232-3472
Juvenile Diabetes Foundation (JDF)
(800) 223-1138

DOCTOR CERTIFICATION
American Board of Medical Specialties
(800) 776-2378

DOWN SYNDROME
National Down Syndrome Congress
(800) 232-NDSC
National Down Syndrome Society
(800) 221-4602

DRUGS
Individuals' Drug-Related Problems
(800) 662-HELP
Just Say No International
(800) 258-2766
National Clearing House
(800) SAY-NOTO
National Drug Information Referral
Line
(800) 662-HELP

DRUGS — DIFFICULT TO LOCATE
National Information Center for
Orphan Drugs and Rare Diseases
(800) 336-4797

DRUGS — FDA
Hotline
(800) 336-4797

DYSLEXIA
Orton Dyslexia Society
(800) ABCD-123

ENDOMETRIOSIS
Endometriosis Assoc.
(800) 992-ENDO

EPILEPSY
Epilepsy Foundation of America
(800) EFA-1000
Epilepsy Information Line
(800) 426-0660

GRIEF RECOVERY
Grief Recovery Helpline
(800) 445-4808

HEAD INJURY
National Head Injury Foundation
(800) 444-6443

HEADACHE
National Headache Foundation
(800) 843-2256

HEALTH FRAUD / COMPLAINTS
Medicare Supplement Marketing
Complaints
(800) 638-6833
National Council Against Health Fraud
(800) 821-6671
Practitioner Reporting System
(to Report Hospitals)
(800) 638-2725
(301) 881-0256 in PA

HEALTH INFORMATION
Consumer Health Information Resource
Institute
(800) 821-6671
U.S. Public Health Service
(800) 336-4797

HEARING
Better Hearing Institute
(800) 424-8576
Deafness Research Foundation
(800) 535-3323

HEARING — Continued
Dial-A-Hearing Test
(800) 222-EARS
(800) 345-EARS in PA
Hearing Helpline
(800) 424-8576
National Assoc. for Hearing and
Speech Action
(800) 638-8255
National Hearing Aid Society
(800) 521-5247
Occupational Hearing Service
(800) 222-3277
Tripod Grapevine
(800) 352-8888

HEART DISEASE
American Heart Assoc.
(800) 242-8721
Assoc. of Heart Patients
(800) 241-6993
Coronary Club, Inc.
No 800 number, write to:
9500 Euclid Ave.
Cleveland, OH 44195
Mended Hearts
No 800 number, write to:
7320 Greenville Ave.
Dallas, TX 75231

HOSPITAL CARE
Hospitals Providing Free Care
(Hill Burton)
(800) 638-0742
(800) 492-0359 in MD
Shriner's Hospital Referral Line
(800) 237-5055
(800) 282-9161 in FL

HUNTINGTON'S DISEASE
Huntington's Disease Society of
America
(800) 345-4372

IMPOTENCE
The Impotence Foundation
(800) 221-5517

INFERTILITY
Resolve
(800) 662-1016

INTESTINES
National Foundation for Ileitis
and Colitis
(800) 343-3637

KIDNEY DISEASE
American Kidney Fund
(800) 638-8299
National Kidney Foundation
(800) 622-9010

LIVER
American Liver Foundation
(800) 223-0179

LUPUS
Lupus Hot Line
(800) 558-0121
Terri Otthelf Lupus Research Institute
(800) 82-LUPUS

MEDICARE
Improper Provider Bill/Service
(800) 368-5779

MENTAL HEALTH
American Mental Health Counselors
Assoc.
(800) 326-2642
American Schizophrenia Assoc.
(800) 783-3801
National Foundation for Depressive
Illness
(800) 248-4344
See Local Listing
Tough Love
Adult Children of Alcoholics
CODA for Co-dependency

MULTIPLE SCLEROSIS
National Multiple Sclerosis Society
(NMSS)
(800) 624-8236

MYASTHENIA GRAVIS
Myasthenia Gravis Foundation
(800) 541-5454

NEUROFIBROMATOSIS
National Neurofibromatosis Foundation
(800) 323-7938

ORGAN DONOR PROGRAMS
The Organ Donor Hot Line
(800) 24-DONOR

OSTEOPATHIC
National Osteopathic Foundation
(NOF)
(800) 621-1773

PARALYSIS
American Paralysis Assoc.
(800) 225-0292

PARKINSON
American Parkinson Disease Assoc.
(800) 223-2732
National Parkinson Foundation
(800) 327-4545
Parkinson's Educational Program USA
(800) 344-7872

PMS
PMS Access
(800) 222-4PMS

PRACTITIONER REPORTING
Practitioner Reporting System
(800) 638-6725
(Reporting of Product Defects)

PRODUCT SAFETY
Consumer Product Safety Commission
(CPSC)
(800) 638-2772

PROSTATE

National Center for Treatment and Research of Prostate Diseases
No 800 number, write to:
Medical College of Wisconsin
Froedtert Memorial
Lutheran Hospital
9200 West Wisconsin Ave.
Milwaukee, WI 53226
National Kidney and Urologic Diseases Information Clearinghouse
No 800 number, write to
(ask for prostatic enlargement brochure):
Box NKUDIC
Bethesda, MD 20892
Prostate Cancer Education Council
No 800 number, write to:
JAF Box 888
New York, NY 10116

RARE DISORDERS

National Organization for Rare Disorders
(800) 999-6673

SHRINERS HOSPITAL

Shriners Hospital Referral Line
(800) 237-5055

SICKLE CELL

National Assoc. for Sickle Cell Disease
(800) 421-8453

SIGHT

American Council of the Blind
(800) 424-8666
American Foundation for the Blind
(800) 232-5463
Blind Children's Center
(800) 222-3566
Contact Lens Manufacturers Assoc.
(800) 343-5367
Guide Dog Foundation for the Blind
(800) 548-4337

SIGHT — Continued

National Alliance of Blind Students
(800) 424-8666
National Eye Care Project
(800) 222-EYES
National Library Services for the Blind and Physically Handicapped
(800) 424-8567
National Retinitis Pigmentosa Foundation
(800) 638-2300
Recording for the Blind (RFB)
(800) 221-4792

SPINA BIFIDA

Spina Bifida Assoc. of America
(800) 621-3141

SPINAL CORD INJURY

National Spinal Cord Injury Assoc.
(800) 962-9629
Spinal Cord Injury National Hot Line
(800) 526-3456

SUICIDE

National Suicide Hot Line
(800) 621-4000

TOURETTE SYNDROME

Tourette Syndrome Assoc. (TSA)
(800) 237-0717

TRANSPLANTS

American Council on Transplantation
(800) ACT-GIVE

TUBEROUS SCLEROSIS

National Tuberous Sclerosis Assoc.
(800) 225-6872

WOMEN'S SPORTS

Women's Sports Foundation
(800) 342-3988

NOTES

Are You Sure...

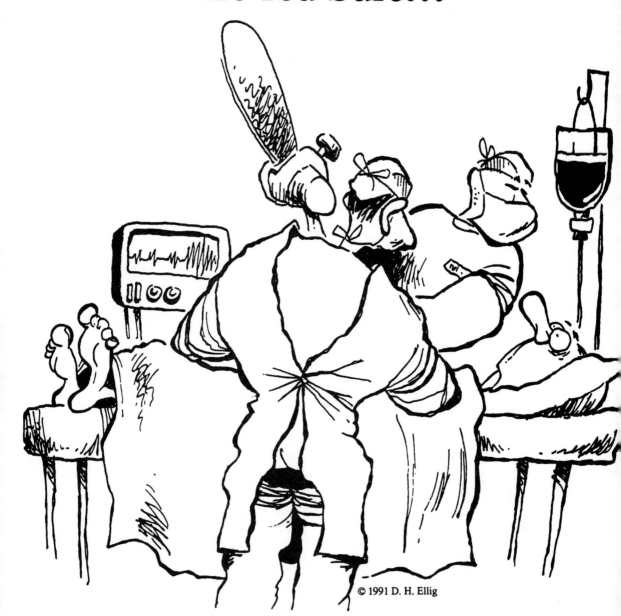

© 1991 D. H. Ellig

You Have Done this Before?

CHAPTER 11

HOW TO QUALIFY HOSPITALS

This chapter contains questions to help you qualify the hospital and to help you feel more relaxed and comfortable during your hospital stay. Whether the treatment is your own or for a loved one, your first visit to a hospital can be bewildering, particularly at a time when you are under high emotional stress. These materials are designed to help you be more fully informed about your treatment plans and rights, so that you may enjoy the world's best medical care.

The majority of medical providers will be more than happy to address the topics in this book. Some won't. Keep in mind that it is always *your* decision to choose who you wish to treat you or a loved one.

You may not use all the suggestions in this chapter. It will depend upon how you entered the hospital, either as an elective entry or as an emergency entry, and what your mental condition is while you are in the hospital. You, a friend or loved one will benefit in many ways by this chapter, even if you only use a small part of it.

If you enter the hospital on an elective basis (most likely since only 5 to 10 percent of hospital admissions are through the emergency room), you have adequate time to research the hospital before your admittance, you may want to address the following issues:

BEFORE CHECK IN THOUGHTS

Precertification

* Have you contacted your insurance company to precertify your hospital stay? If not, it might not cover all the charges.

Preferred Providers

* If your program has preferred providers (PPO), have you confirmed that all the professionals providing services are PPO providers?

    Many medical plans now have different payment schedules for PPO and non-PPO providers. If you use non-PPO providers, your cost for medical services could increase. Therefore, it is beneficial to check to see if the hospital, labs and all the doctors providing services are PPO providers.

    If some providers are non-PPO providers, you might want to discuss this with your primary physician and to ask the non-PPO providers if the insurance company's payment will be accepted in full, or will they waive excessive fees.

Second Opinion

* Does your insurance company require a second opinion for your medical procedure?

    If it does and you didn't obtain a second opinion, it might not cover all charges and your share of the cost could be greater.

Outpatient Option

* Are you sure your hospital stay is necessary? Or can your procedure be safely done on an outpatient basis?

    If your insurance company requires some procedures to be performed as outpatient only, if one of these procedures is done inpatient, you may have to pay the difference.

Ask Your Doctor

* Have you discussed the questions suggested in "Ask Your Doctor" with your medical provider?

You may want to tape record the conversation with your doctor concerning procedure description, risk factors, success rates (or doctor's definition of success), recovery rates and time frame, and the patient's responsibility to help speed the recovery process.

If there is any doubt regarding any of these issues, you might want to request documented cases or studies.

Morning Admission Option

* Can you schedule your admittance in the morning rather than the night before?

A morning admittance will not only reduce the cost of your hospital stay, but enable you to be more rested and relaxed by sleeping at your own home, versus a strange hospital setting.

Preadmission Tests

* Have you had your preadmission testing before you entered the hospital? Did you confirm that all the tests were necessary? Did you research the testing accuracy rate of the lab?

Location of Hospital

* Is the hospital close to you or close to your doctor? Do you have a choice?

Occasionally doctors have admitting privileges at several hospitals. Some hospitals provide doctors free or discounted office space at the hospital and occasionally provide financial aide to doctors. You may want to understand why the doctor is recommending this particular hospital and if the hospital has contributed financial aide or office space to your doctor.

It may also be appropriate to ask the doctor's help to get access to the hospital's quality information. If the doctor is referring you to a particular hospital, he should be aware of these values, have the information available or assist you in getting hospital quality information (discussed in later chapters).

QUALITY ISSUES

Hospital Accreditation Rating

* Have you checked the hospital accreditation with the Joint Commission on Accreditation of Health Care Organizations (JCAHO) 312/642-6061, 857 N. Michigan Ave., Chicago, IL 60611. The hospital will be rated as accredited (84 to 90%), conditional accreditation (5 to 8%) or not accredited (1 to 2%). Since most hospitals have passed the accreditation process, there should be no reason for you to visit a hospital that hasn't passed. Check with your doctor if you have any questions.

Radiology Accreditation

* Is your radiology department accredited by the American College of Radiology (ACR)?

    Accreditation by the American College of Radiology means that the radiology staff and equipment have passed certain criteria.

Usually hospitals are not accustomed to prospective patients asking the next three questions and may offer some resistance. The front desk staff may not have the information but the administrative offices do. If there is resistance, try asking for help from the hospital administrator or your referring doctor as it should be his responsibility to select the best quality providers.

Board Certified Specialists

* Have you compared the number of doctors with admitting privileges to the number of doctors who are Board *certified* (as opposed to Board *qualified*)?

    Studies indicate that mortality rates are lower at hospitals with a higher percentage of Board certified specialists than hospitals with lower percentages. Most hospitals should have 75 to 80 percent of their doctors board certified.

Registered Nurses

* Have you compared the percentage of Registered Nurses at this hospital with the ratio at other hospitals?

    Studies indicate that patient outcomes are better at hospitals that have a higher percentage of Registered Nurses than at hospitals that have a low percentage.

Occupancy Rate

* Have you compared the occupancy rate of this hospital with the occupancy rate at other hospitals?

Hospital occupancy rates can be an indication of patient outcome. The higher the occupancy the better the outcome. The average hospital occupancy rate in the United States is 58 percent, however, some cities may have a 100 percent occupancy rate.

Additionally, the occupancy rate may correlate with the cost. The lower the occupancy rate the higher the cost because more revenues must be generated to cover the cost of the empty beds.

Hospital Infection Rate

* Have you compared the hospital-caused infection (nosocomial) rate with the infection rate at other hospitals?

This will probably be a very difficult question for the hospital staff to answer, but you can understand the importance of asking it. Because of its importance, make an extra effort to get this information. **It _is_ available.**

Infection control is an important issue. The National Foundation of Infections Disease estimates 2 million patients are infected while in the hospital at an annual cost of $2.8 billion — that is billion — not million.

If the hospital is reviewed by JCAHO (Joint Commission on Accreditation of Health Care Organizations), it is required to track and document their infection control efforts. The hospital has the data.

Hospital Mortality Rate

* Have you compared the mortality rate at this hospital with the mortality rate at other hospitals?

A detailed report containing the accreditation data, and infection and mortality rates may be available from your State Department of Health, Licensing Division. If not, the Federal Department of Health Care Financing Administration may have a copy. These reports will show the infection and mortality rates. They however are very difficult to read and interpret.

This may be difficult for you to obtain. It _is_ available and you have a right to have this information. Many times hospitals with high mortality rates will suggest the rate is high because they handle the most complicated cases. If this is the case, ask for documentation supporting that statement. Do not simply accept the statement. Ask them to prove it. Sometimes this question may be difficult for hospitals to answer because they believe high mortality rates are caused by the type of patients they treat, not hospital administrative controls.

All hospitals carry medical malpractice insurance. Most medical malpractice insurance companies provide the hospitals with a "loss" run report that shows what kind of claim, where it happened, and what caused the claim. Hospitals and insurance companies use this report to identify the risks and suggest ways to reduce them. A hospital should know where their problems are. The public may experience difficulty getting the information, however.

If the hospital is reluctant to provide this information, you may want to ask your doctor for his help. If he is referring you to a particular hospital, he should be aware of the information, have it available or request that the hospital provide you with this data.

Procedure Frequency

* Have you checked the number of times your specific procedure has been performed at this hospital? Do other hospitals perform it more or less?

Studies indicate that the more times a procedure is performed, the lower the mortality and complication rates. Lowest rates occur when procedure is performed over 350 times per year. Highest rates occur when procedure is performed less than 200 times per year.

Staff Drug Testing Program

* Does the hospital have a drug testing program for members of the surgical team or nursing staff?

Many firms in the United States have implemented drug testing programs for their employees. Surprisingly, very few hospitals have implemented drug and alcohol testing programs.

It would seem that the hospital would want the public to know the surgical team responsible for the successful outcome in life and death situations was operating at its best, without impairment. Wouldn't it be nice if hospitals had a drug and alcohol testing program for professionals practicing at their facility? Wouldn't it be nice if the public demanded it? Yet, as of this printing, only one hospital (John Hopkins) has considered implementing a drug and alcohol testing policy for the doctors and surgical staff. The already accredited doctors felt this was unnecessary and an infringement of their rights. Apparently their rights are more important than the patient's, as now John Hopkins is considering testing only new doctors and only once, when they are first credentialed.

Nutrition Support Team

* Does the hospital have a nutrition support team that monitors your *specific* nutrient requirements and intake? Who is on the team (registered dietician, pharmacist, specialist doctor and nurse)? Do they monitor your charts/treatment?

    As simple as this question sounds, studies show that if an individual is hospitalized for more than five days, many times it is possible to suffer a nutritional deficiency or, in extreme cases, malnourishment. Therefore, it is important that the hospital staff have a nutrition support team to continually monitor your specific requirements, particularly if you will be having an extended hospital stay.

    If a patient suffers a 10 percent or greater weight loss while hospitalized, patient nutrient intake should be monitored.

Bioethics Team

* Does the hospital have a bioethics consulting team?

    Bioethic consulting is a team that provides support information for those who must make the decision of whether to continue use of life support systems. The team usually consists of a staff doctor, the primary care physician, a nurse, a social worker and a minister. They provide the decision maker with the options available, technical data, possible outcomes and prognosis. It truly is a support group so the decision maker can make an informed decision. It will help relieve the stress of the decision.

    A bioethics consulting team is a new service and very few hospitals will have a team available, but there will be more.

Reference Check

* Have you called your State Board of Medical Examiners or American Medical Association to check *all doctors involved* (surgeon, assistant surgeon, anesthesiologist or Certified Registered Nurse Anesthetist) for complaints, license revocation, etc.?

    *This experience may not be the same as dealing with the Better Business Bureau. A telephone call might not help you obtain the information you want or need. You might have to schedule an appointment with the Board office, appear in person, and sign the doctor's file stating you had access to his records. If you are not in the same town as the Board of Medical Examiners, you might have to make your request in writing and pay copying costs. (Generally the Board **does not allow files to be copied**).*

If you have difficulty getting this information, ask your referring physician for help. Since he is referring you to these doctors, he should know the answers. You may also want to document his response on the "Informed Consent Checklist" shown in the chapter on consent forms.

Do not assume that if a doctor is admitted to practice at a hospital that his record is clean. It is possible for a doctor to have a poor record in one state and simply move his practice to another state.

Hospitals try to deny staff credentials to doctors they know have questionable records, but will give the doctor admitting and treatment privileges because of fear of restraint of trade lawsuits from a denied doctor. (Fifty percent of insurance liability claims filed against hospitals by physicians and allied health professionals involve credentialing issues.) Every hospital administrator has at one time or another been forced to credential a physician whose poor record caused the hospital administrator concern.

Unfortunately, many times it becomes the patient's responsibility to determine physician quality, because the physician and hospital communities may be afraid to make quality statements out of fear of litigation.

COST ISSUES

Cost Comparison

* Have you compared the costs (room and ancillary charges) at this hospital with other hospitals?

   (Some State Health Departments make public cost comparisons of *specific procedures* available to the public.)

Doctor's Admitting and Release Fee

* Will there be a doctor's admitting fee? Why should you have to pay if he's not present at admitting?

* Will there be a doctor's release fee? Why should you pay if he's not present at the time of release?

   The AMA *Principles of Medical Ethics* states that an administrative fee to admit a patient to the hospital is unethical.

ANESTHESIOLOGY

Meeting Your Anesthesiologist

*   Have you met your anesthesiologist?

    Very few patients ever meet their anesthesiologist until they are about to be anesthetized. This is the wrong time to discuss his qualifications and the type of anesthesia you wish. (See Chapter 6, "Ask Your Doctor," to learn how to qualify.)

Certified Registered Nurse Anesthetist

*   Does the hospital allow your anesthesia to be monitored and controlled by a Certified Registered Nurse Anesthetist (CRNA) under the direction of an M.D.?

    Some states allow a Certified Registered Nurse Anesthetist to perform the task of the anesthesiologist under the direction of the anesthesiologist. "Under the direction" normally means that the anesthesiologist must be on-site, but not necessarily in the room. If you feel uncomfortable about the use of a Certified Registered Nurse Anesthetist, you will want to discuss this with your doctor.

*   How many CRNA's may the anesthesiologist direct at one time?

    If there are more than two you might want to discuss this with your doctor, as the anesthesiologist can only handle one problem at a time.

Type of Anesthesia

*   Have you discussed what type of anesthesia will be used — general/local — and how will it be administered? by gas/injection/IV? Have the risks versus the benefits of each type/method been explained to you?

    Anesthesia may be administered by four broad methods:

    Local Block — The anesthesia only affects a limited area of the body. An example of this is the Novocain administered by a dentist. An anesthesiologist need not be present to administer this type of anesthesia.

    Regional Block — This anesthesia affects a whole region of the body, but the brain is not affected and you do not lose consciousness.

    The advantage to the first two is that the patient is conscious and can communicate with the doctor and the anesthesiologist during the operation.

General Anesthesia — This anesthesia causes the patient to be unconscious and not be able to communicate with the physicians. You only regain consciousness when the anesthesia wears off or an antidote is applied.

General Anesthesia with Intubation — This type of anesthesia not only causes the patient to be unconscious but also paralyzed. It requires other physicians and machines to keep the important body functions operating. This procedure requires a tube be placed in the patient's mouth and throat.

Safe Anesthesia

* Have you informed the anesthesiologist that you want to have the least toxic anesthesia?

Usually a local anesthesia is less toxic and therefore less dangerous.

OTHER QUESTIONS

Cell Research

* Does the hospital or your doctor participate in commercial or scientific cell research?

Recently there has been much dispute regarding patient cell ownership. In a recent case, a patient's cells were used to develop an anticancer drug.

The patient stated he had not been informed that his cells were to be used for research and requested royalties. The market for the drug was estimated to exceed $3 billion and the doctor would profit from the sale. At this time, the case is being litigated.

If it is important to you to know if your cells will be used for research, you will want to discuss this with your physician.

Blood Donation

* If your surgical procedure requires you to need blood, have you previously donated your own?

Scientific studies indicate that the *best blood* to use during a surgical procedure *is your own*. Your own blood will reduce the risk of complications and increase the chances of a quicker recovery. Normally you may donate a pint a week for four weeks before your surgery, another reason to discuss if surgery can be delayed. If you cannot use your own blood, discuss with your doctor other means of possibly reducing the amount of donated blood.

Do Not Resuscitate Orders

*   Have you asked about the hospital's policy regarding "Do Not Resuscitate" (DNR) orders?

DNR orders outline the extent to which hospital staff are to apply lifesaving or life-recovery procedures, i.e., don't try or try to the utmost.

This important issue will have to be addressed at check in. You should know the hospital's policy before you schedule your admission. If the hospital is accredited by the Joint Commission on Accreditation of Health Care Organizations, it will have this policy since it is a part of the accreditation process.

Once you have read the hospital's DNR policy, you may want to discuss it with your physician and determine his attitude and yours regarding this policy.

Medical Database Access

*   Does the hospital have access to the National Library of Medicine Databases such as MEDLINE, PDQ and others for latest treatment plans? Does your physician use it?

MEDLINE is the largest database containing bibliographic data from over 3,500 medical journals. It is frequently used to research what treatments are available and the expected outcomes.

PDQ is a reference source database maintained by the National Cancer Institute and has four files:

1)   State of the art cancer information
2)   A doctor directory
3)   An organization directory
4)   Cancer protocols

Hospital Medical Library

*   In order to provide you with details about your condition/treatment plans/risks, may you have access to the hospital medical library to review medical books and databases, journals and studies?

Visitors

* Is it possible to arrange to have a loved one, family or friend share your room and meals with you during your hospital stay?

    This question should definitely be asked if you have a child receiving in-hospital treatment. You should ascertain if you may stay with that child on a 24-hour basis so that you can monitor care and provide comfort.

    If you cannot stay with the child on a 24-hour basis because of other obligations, you should ask the child to call you (if he is old enough) if there are any changes in his treatment or testing procedures.

    You should also inform the doctor and hospital staff that they should discuss these changes with you thoroughly before implementing.

Meals

* Is it possible for family members to bring meals from home to the patient?

    Many hospitals now allow loved ones to remain overnight with the patient and to bring home cooked meals (within guidelines) to the patient. The patient's hospital stay can be less stressful when maintaining contact with family and the home environment.

Hospital Tour

* Have you toured the hospital to look at the rooms and facilities?

COMPARISON OF HOSPITAL
QUALITY AND SERVICE ISSUES

	HOSPITAL 1	HOSPITAL 2
Preferred Provider (PPO)		
Accredited by JACHO		
Accredited by ACR		
Infection Rate		
Complication Rate		
Mortality Rate		
Percent of ABMS Board Certified Doctors		
Percent of Registered Nurses		
Occupancy Rate		
Provides Price Estimates		
Performed Procedure _____ Times		
Certified "Drug Free" Doctors and Staff		
Certified "AIDS Free" Doctors and Staff		
Nutrition Support Team		
Bioethics Consulting Team		
Free Access to Medical Library/Databases		
Provides Copies of Medical Records		
Lab Testing Accuracy		
Tested by What Organizations		
Location of Hospital		
Facility Appearance		

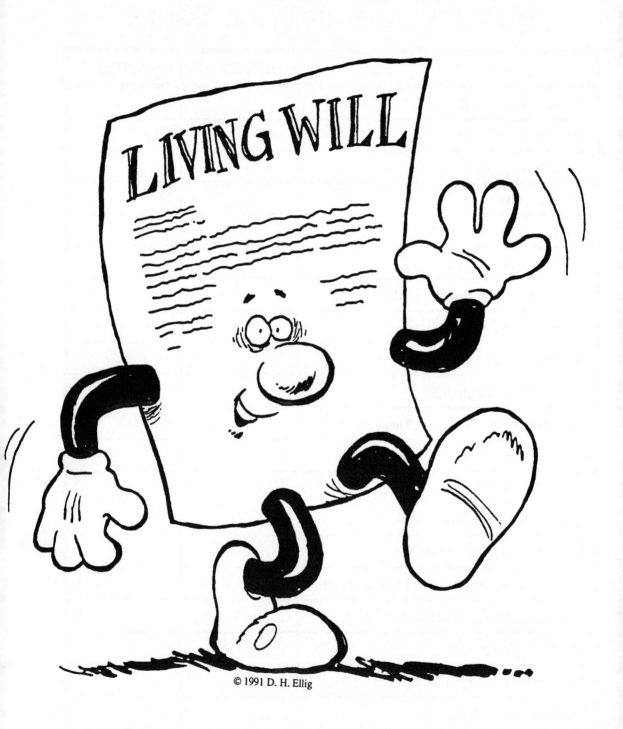

© 1991 D. H. Ellig

CHAPTER 12

LIVING WILL

One of the issues you will have to address when you are admitted to the hospital is the Living Will or Medical Power of Attorney. It is best to understand the Living Will concept before you are confronted with 15 different admitting forms.

It is estimated that only 15 percent of the United States population has a Living Will or Durable Power of Attorney, documents that allow a patient to refuse future medical treatment while he is still of sound mind and body. A recent Supreme Court decision illustrates the need to place your wishes in writing concerning any future medical treatment you might need.

WHY IT IS NEEDED

The United States Supreme Court has ruled that *verbally* stated wishes to refuse medical treatment which unnecessarily prolong life are not legally binding unless there is "clear and convincing" evidence of such wishes. If you have told a friend or loved one that you do not want to continue to live as a vegetable and expect that wish to be carried out, it won't and can't happen based on this Supreme Court ruling.

The premise of the Living Will is based on the fact that while you are conscious and functioning normally, you have the legal right to accept or reject medical treatment. This document allows you to place your feelings in writing about future medical treatment if you become unconscious or mentally incapacitated from a sudden, unexpected accident or illness.

While this chapter is titled "Living Will" there are other names for documents that address the issues discussed in the chapter. Your state may have laws that dictate which form to use. It is best to check with a hospital, healthcare professional or legal counsel before preparing a Living Will. The New Patient Self-determination Act requires hospitals to inform patients of their right to refuse medical services and to provide patients a written description of the state law.

The names for these documents are

Living Will

Healthcare Power of Attorney

Durable Power of Attorney

Durable Medical Power of Attorney

Durable General Power of Attorney

You need to be sure that the document will be effective if you are *either terminally ill* or *incompetent.* Many older documents were effective only if your medical condition was terminal. It is possible to be incompetent and not terminally ill, i.e., people living in a vegetative state for years. It is estimated by some sources that hospitals have 10,000 patients living in a permanent vegetative state, without being terminal.

The "Patient Self-Determination Act" (effective December 1991) requires healthcare providers that provide services for Medicare and Medicaid patients to furnish information about the use of a Living Will or Healthcare Power of Attorney. Most hospital admitting forms will have a section for the patient to express their wishes.

WHAT IT DOES

The documents will protect you from a lengthy period of pain and suffering, avoid heartache and stress for your loved ones, reduce the chance of your estate being depleted or, worse yet, create a large debt for your loved ones.

The Living Will can preserve your estate from the ravages of high medical costs or save your loved ones from large debts. The document should state that the decision to refuse treatment will be based upon competent medical evidence.

You can designate a person to act on your behalf in the event that you do not fully recover from surgery or treatment. The document will protect the designated person who acts on your behalf and adheres to your wishes if you become unconscious or mentally incapacitated from a catastrophic medical condition.

The document may state that you do not fear death as much as the indignity of deterioration, dependency and hopeless pain.

The Living Will should state that if the only purpose of heroic medical effort is to postpone the moment of death because your body is substantially damaged, deteriorated or in tenuous medical condition through accident, illness or age and there is no reasonable expectation of recovery from physical or mental disability, the effort should be stopped. You may state that you expect withdrawal of life-prolonging means and measures, so that you may die with dignity and lessen the suffering of loved ones.

The document normally may have to be notarized and witnessed and should be given to your doctor and the hospital when you check in.

ISSUES TO BE ADDRESSED

Who will be your agent?

Be sure to appoint someone you know and trust to carry out your wishes. Healthcare providers are normally not appropriate and some states prohibit them from acting as your agent.

Effective Date of Agent's Power

Your document should state when the agent can start to make medical care decisions on your behalf, terminally ill, incompetent or during periods of incapacity. Normally, the decision when to invoke the agent's power of attorney is made jointly with your physician and your agent. It is important that they both understand your wishes clearly.

Agent Powers

These are normally limited to healthcare decisions. You may make them very broad or you can restrict them to only certain issues.

Generally the agent's powers are the same as the powers you would have, but it is best to clarify the following issues:

Directive to withhold or withdraw:
— Medical treatment
— Maximum life prolonging treatment
— Nutrition (food) and hydration (water) treatment
— Directive to make medical care decisions such as treatment, tests, drugs, access to medical records, hospital discharge, etc.

Sources for Copies

As of the printing of this book, Living Wills were acceptable in 39 states. In those states without Living Will laws, you may use a generalized statement of your wishes with a Durable Power of Attorney for healthcare that names a third party as an agent of your wishes. All states have laws allowing power of attorney and most have laws specifying how the power of attorney should be configured specifically for healthcare. For specific information respecting your state and examples of legal documents, contact one of the sources at the end of this chapter.

There are many preprinted copies of Living Will forms available from office supply stores, stationery stores, nursing homes, and possibly, medical providers. They are rather inexpensive, ranging from $1.00 to $5.00. Your attorney can also draft one for you (estimated cost is $80 - $300 per document).

An up-to-date source of a Living Will or a Durable Power of Attorney for healthcare in your state of residence can be secured from the following:

AARP Fulfillment, Request: Healthcare Powers of Attorney, 1909 K Street N.W., Washington, DC 20049

Society for the Right to Die, Request "Living Will Example," 250 W. 57th Street, New York, NY 10107

National Hemlock Society, P.O. Box 11830, Eugene, OR 97440

Generally, all of these organizations provide up-to-date forms that include the most recent wording reflected by state and federal laws.

NOTES

Too Late To Ask Questions!

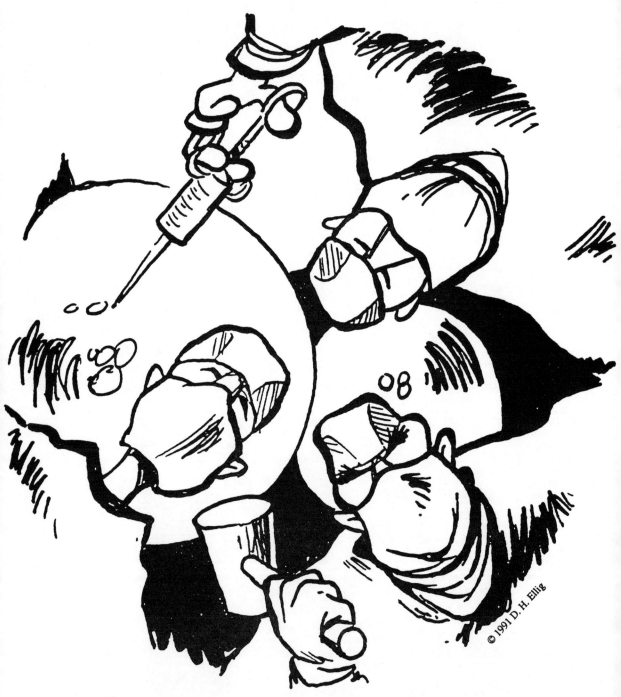

Ah, About Your Qualifications...

CHAPTER 13

HOSPITAL CHECK IN QUESTIONS

At check in you will be presented with many forms to sign. Hospitals generally refer to these as "informed consent forms," however, they more resemble "uninformed consent forms" and do more to protect the hospital than the patient. They provide the hospital great latitude to perform procedures and practices without your consent (i.e., when you are under anesthesia). Review the forms carefully to be sure that you don't sign away your rights or authorize procedures you do not wish or about which you have not been informed. The chapter on consent forms discussed some of the issues which will be covered in detail in this chapter.

It is best to resolve consent issues during the check in process. It is very difficult, if not impossible, to do so after you have signed all the forms. Even if you inadvertently sign away some of your rights, please be aware you cannot sign away the hospital's liability.

Remember, this is your last chance to retain control of what will happen to you or your loved ones.

CONSENT FORM CHANGES

Consent Forms

* Did you review the hospital consent form and cross out any "open-ended" treatment statements?

157

Expect to have some lively discussions regarding your changes with the hospital staff. If you are having difficulties, ask to discuss these difficulties with management-level personnel or the hospital administrator. Very few patients take the initiative to carefully review and cross out open-ended treatment statements that allow the doctor to perform any additional surgery he feels is appropriate. Failure to define procedures and expectations beforehand may result in the medical team performing medical procedures you do not authorize or want.

* You may want to amend or add to the hospital consent form with the following:

a.   You will consent to the surgery only if your doctor performs the surgery and only if assisted by those doctors you have already approved and listed by name.

Occasionally doctors will admit patients and, for many different reasons, turn the surgery over to another physician. If you have taken an active part in your treatment as discussed in this book, you will probably feel uncomfortable with a switch in doctors at the last minute. Your amended consent note, specifying your choice in physicians, will notify the doctor and hospital of your desires.

b.   You authorize only the procedure previously discussed with your doctor.

Many times the hospital consent form allows the physician to perform other procedures based on his judgment at the time of surgery. This clause normally contains words such as "can perform whatever additional surgery is deemed necessary." If you feel uncomfortable with this and would like to discuss additional surgeries before they are performed, you should strike this clause and note that you prefer to discuss additional surgeries before they are performed.

c.   If you have any reservations about the treatment plan, note them on the consent form.

d.   Do you want your operation observed or recorded for educational purposes? If not, state so in writing on the hospital consent form.

e.   May a loved one, family member or friend observe the operation?

This may be the first time the hospital has received such an inquiry. Your chances of receiving an affirmative response are very slim, but for those of your family members or friends who would like to be present, it is worth making the request.

As an example of hospital policy changes, for many years fathers were not allowed in delivery rooms and now it is very common.

If you are present at a loved one's operation, you will know what is happening when it happens and relieve you of that terrible waiting period.

An additional benefit is that human nature is such that the quality of work improves when it is being observed by an interested person. Could also be true of physicians and hospital staff?

f. Do you want to relinquish your rights to future experiments or commercial sale of your cells, tissues or organs which might be removed during the operation?

Now is the time to put your desires regarding possible sale or profit from your cells, tissues or organs in writing.

g. Did you state that you want to be informed of all test results?

Many times test results are not provided to the patient by the doctor's order. As an informed patient, if you want to know test results, now is the time to place your request in writing. Without this request, test results could be withheld from you.

The results of a pathology report is a good example. It will provide you with the results of any testing outcomes, normal or abnormal. Hospitals do not operate like your local garage. They do not return the damaged parts! You need the pathology report to determine if the part was damaged.

h. If you want access to your medical records, have you stated it in writing?

Your medical records might legally be yours depending on state law. You might however be charged for copies. Your records may be released to anyone you choose.

With our increasing mobile society, it is becoming more important for patients to compile a medical records file that can provide a new doctor in a new city vital past medical history information.

Heroic Effort

*   Did you indicate in writing your definition of "heroic effort," such as resuscitation, CPR, respirator, IV? Does it conflict with the hospital's Do Not Resuscitate (DNR) Policy?

As an example, if hospital DNR policy states they must try their utmost lifesaving and life-recovery procedures to prolong your life and your Living Will instruction conflicts with hospital policy — your wishes are no "heroic effort" — how will you handle it? (See section on Living Will for more detail.)

Organ Donation

*   Do you wish to donate your organs to science or people?

     If so, specify it in writing.

     If you are not satisfied with the conditions listed on the hospital consent forms, you may sign the forms with a note of reservation, indicating that signing the consent form was a condition of admittance.

OTHER FORMS

Patient's Bill of Rights

*   Did you receive a copy of your "Patient's Bill of Rights"?

     If the hospital receives any federal funds, such as Medicare, they are required to provide you with a copy of the "Patient's Bill of Rights."

Living Will

*   Did you provide a notarized copy of your Living Will to be placed in your hospital admitting file? (See section on Living Will for more detail.)

     The Patient Self-Determination Act requires hospitals to advise patients of their right to sign advance instructions (Living Will or Health Care Power of Attorney) for healthcare in the event of incapacity and a written description of state law. Most hospital admittance forms will have a section for the patient to note their desires.

OTHER QUESTIONS

Hospital Bill

*   Did you request an itemized bill so you can compare it with your log of services recorded on the service log form? (See example at end of this chapter.)

*   Did you request the itemized bill in layman's terms you are able to understand? (Example: aspirin, not acetylsalicylic acid. It is easier for the hospital to charge $2.00 for a tablet of acetylsalicylic acid which the patient doesn't understand than $2.00 for an aspirin tablet.)

Patient Advocate

*   Do you know the name and telephone number of your patient advocate (the person at the hospital who will assist you with hospital policy and rights)?

Life Insurance and Cobeneficiary

*   Do any of the forms suggest that the hospital will be cobeneficiary on your life insurance policy?

    Very few hospitals now have this policy. In the past, however, some hospitals did request to be a cobeneficiary on life insurance policies as a means of ensuring payment of the hospital bill.

SHARING IS NICE

But, please wash your hands...

I am sick enough.

CHAPTER 14

IN-HOSPITAL QUESTIONS

Hospitals, which are established to heal the sick, are actually not healthy places to stay. It is possible to acquire an illness while you are in the hospital because of other patients' illnesses and your weakened condition. Some studies have indicated that 20 percent to 30 percent of patients who enter the hospital acquire hospital-caused infections [nosocomial] that could produce complications and result in longer hospital stays or death. If the national hospital infection rate for hospital-caused infections was only 10 percent, it is estimated that 100,000 deaths per year could occur.

AVOID UNNECESSARY INFECTION

The **simplest** way to reduce your chances of acquiring a hospital caused infection is to post a sign requesting all hospital personnel to wash their hands in your presence before touching you, your personal items or your bedding. The staff might voice objections, but you have the right to control your life and your body. It is estimated that without your reminder to wash their hands, hospital staff will follow the hand washing guidelines only 40 percent of the time.

If the staff are wearing rubber gloves, ask your care giver to change into a fresh pair. A used pair of rubber gloves protects only the care giver, not the patient. Since the infection-causing agent is **on** the glove, *it could be on you.*

EXERCISE YOUR RIGHTS

Doctor's Orders

* Have you discussed with your doctor your wish to be fully informed and involved in any treatment performed? Has he informed the hospital staff of your wishes? Has he noted your wishes on your chart? (Doctor's orders — "Patient wants to be informed — answer all questions.")

Drugs

* Tell your doctor you want to know what drugs are prescribed, what dosages and how often. Write it down so you can monitor the drugs that are given to you. Studies show that hospitals may have a 3 percent to 20 percent dispensing error. You can make sure that you are not in the 3 percent to 20 percent group.

Physician's Desk Reference

* If you are given medication, you may request a copy of the *Physician's Desk Reference* (PDR) (normally available at the nursing station) which lists dosage recommendations according to age and weight, possible reactions, side effects or multiple drug interactions.

    Use of the *Physician's Desk Reference (PDR)* will inform you about drug side effects. You will be able to determine whether the symptoms you are experiencing are a result of illness or surgery, or a drug side effect. Your concerns can be eased by knowing you are experiencing a drug side effect rather than a surgical complication.

    Occasionally, medications and dosages are misdirected to the patient. The PDR can also confirm that you are receiving the right medication and the correct dosage.

Testing

* If you are bothered by the amount of testing being performed, ask why each test is necessary. If there is a retest, ask why the retest is necessary.

    It may be necessary for two different hospital departments to perform tests based on your samples. Rather than provide two separate samples at two different times, why not arrange to provide a larger sample or ask that the departments share the sample. If the retest is due to mishandling of the sample, ask if you will be billed for the second test and why.

Know Your Doctor

*   If you don't know the doctor attending to you, you may refuse to discuss your treatment with him or her.

Teaching Hospitals

*   If you are admitted in a teaching hospital, you should try to ascertain whether you are discussing your care with a doctor, a resident doctor, intern or a student. You can, of course, insist that you discuss your condition with only your doctor.

    If you discuss your condition with anyone other than your admitting doctor, particularly if the doctor is an intern or student, you might want to be a very active participant. The intern or student is in training and may be working exceptionally long hours which can impair his judgment (some shifts last 36 hours on, 12 hours off).

    While in the hospital, keep in mind that anytime you speak with a doctor, even in response to the doctor's question, "How are you doing?" you or your insurance company could be billed for a hospital visit.

Service Dissatisfaction

*   If you are dissatisfied with treatment, services or answers to your questions, call the hospital Patient Advocate for assistance, or you may complain directly to the hospital administrator.

Discharging Yourself

*   If you are dissatisfied with medical treatment or services, you may check out of the hospital against medical advice (AMA) without signing any forms. This could, however, relieve the hospital of any liability for future consequences.

    The hospital staff will normally advise against discharging yourself, suggesting that by discharging yourself you are relieving them of any liability. That may or may not be true, but normally the reason patients discharge themselves against medical advice is because they have changed their mind or are dissatisfied with the treatment plan or services provided.

    You may discharge yourself, but it should be carefully thought through. Other medical care should be arranged before the discharge.

WHEN YOU GET OUT

Room Charges

*   Do you know the time of day room charges begin? May you check out before the start of the new day charge?

    Much like hotels and motels, many hospitals identify a certain hour of the day as the start of a new billing day. If you are discharged even ten minutes after the beginning of that billing day, you or your insurance company could be charged for a full day. Therefore when you are involved in your discharge planning, you should take the start of the new billing day into consideration.

Hospital-acquired Infection

*   Was your stay extended because of a hospital-acquired infection (nosocomial)? Will you have to pay for the extended stay? Why?

    One of the unique features of the medical services delivery system is that we, as consumers, normally do not challenge the additional cost of either treatment error or hospital-acquired infections. If we take our car to a garage and they replace the wrong part or damage additional parts while working, we would strenuously challenge the additional charges. Yet, very few of us challenge additional hospital charges. Why? Because most of us view the hospital bill as the insurance company's expense, when in fact it is our own.

    If we want medical insurance to be affordable, we must challenge inappropriate billing.

Billed for Hospital Errors

*   Did you receive medication or treatment in error? Were you billed for those services? Will you have to pay? Why?

    Sometimes hospitals will provide treatment not ordered by the doctor or will redo tests because the staff made a mistake or gave the patient the wrong medications. Check the bill to see if you are billed for their mistakes.

Hospital Discharge and Payment

*   Are you required to pay your share of the hospital bill before you are discharged?

    Dispute over the patient's share of the bill is one of the issues that commonly arises at discharge. Some hospital billing departments might suggest that you may not be discharged until your share of the bill has been paid. This, of course, is simply not true. If confronted with this situation, simply ask to use a phone to call either an attorney or a local law enforcement branch to notify them that you or your loved one is being held for money (a portion of the bill). You will probably be allowed to leave the hospital without paying your share until the insurance company has paid its portion of your claim.

If it is suggested that you use a credit card to assure payment, be careful. Not only may it be more difficult to resolve disputed charges (both the hospital and doctors), but it may take longer and you will have to pay 16 to 20 percent interest on charges. If you do use a charge card, protect yourself by noting on the charge slip "only **covered reasonable charges** to a **maximum** of **'x' dollars** may be billed."

Medical Records

* Did you leave with a copy of your medical records?

    Now is the time to ask for your medical records if you haven't already. Hospitals cannot hold your records for "ransom," i.e., not release them until the bill has been paid.

Implant Information

* If you had implant surgery (a manufactured part such as joints, lenses, valves, etc.), write a certified letter to the manufacturer requesting to be placed on the notification list for recalls, warnings, product improvements, etc. Think of the letter as your way of registering the warranty. We register the warranty for many consumer products such as TVs, VCRs and toasters. Why not implant devices? (Do you suppose medical device manufacturers have warranties to protect the consumer against manufacturing defects? Have you seen one? Seems like a good idea.)

    Most manufacturers only notify doctors of recalls, warnings and improvements. Therefore, if you are not in contact with your doctor, you could be in a life-threatening position if the implant has been recalled or a warning notice has been issued.

    A real life example of this problem occurred when a heart valve was found to be possibly defective. After three years of trying to contact 23,000 patients who had a possible life-threatening valve installed, only 5,560 of patients had been contacted, despite a nationwide search and notification in newspapers. Don't let it happen to you! You should call 1-800-245-1492 if you had a Bjork-Shiley Convexo-Concave (C-C) heart valve implanted from 1976 through 1986, as the strut may fracture.

Did you know that 25 to 50 medical devices have been recalled in the past ten years, involving 300,000 plus patients?

For a $25 fee the International Implant Registry will register your implant in their database. They monitor warnings and recalls published by the FDA and if your device appears on the FDA list they will notify you. Their number is 1-800-344-3226.

If you receive a recall notice from the manufacturer, be sure to check with your current medical advisor before taking any action.

Continuing Care

* Have you discussed your continuing care plans after discharge with your doctor and hospital staff?

* What is expected of me?

You should make sure you clearly understand how to take your medication, how often, and if you have to continue taking your medication even after you start to feel better.

You should understand when to call your doctor, such as what changes or signs which would require a call to the doctor. You should know when you can expect to start feeling better.

Do you know if you have to change your diet, start exercising? How much rest is expected.

Self-Help Groups

* If you have a serious illness, have you received a list of community self-help programs and telephone numbers?

A list of support groups and contacts is also available in the chapter on support groups.

Send a Card

* If you received outstanding care from a particular individual or group you should send a short thank you note. People want to know they did a good job and that their work was appreciated.

Reorder from: MED. ED. INC., P.O. Box 40696, Mesa, Arizona 85274-0496

HOSPITAL SERVICE LOG

Below is a form which may be used to record all items brought into your room (ordered or not ordered, correct or incorrect, telephone calls, tests, medication whether they're pills, shots, or IV's, doctor visits, nurse visits, and any dispensed items). Remember, you will be charged for everything that enters your room!!!

This form can also be used to record your test results and your temperature and blood pressure readings.

This will provide you with a written record of the level and type of service you received which may be used at a later date to audit your bill, if you so desire.

Date	Time	Service	Est. Cost	Who	Why	Refused	Dosage

Watch Out For The Bill

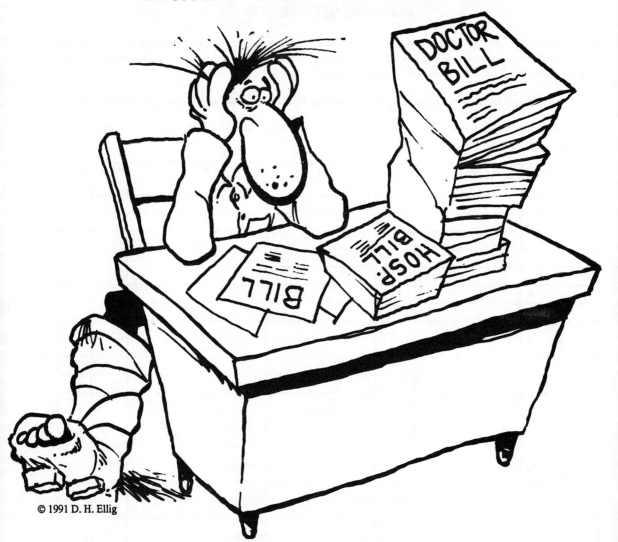

© 1991 D. H. Ellig

But They Said,
"Don't Worry, Your Insurance Will Cover It!"

CHAPTER 15

WATCH OUT FOR THE BILL!

Many times patients and doctors assume that because the patient has medical insurance all charges for services provided will be paid by their insurance company. **This is not true!!**

All insurance contracts have limits as to what services will be covered and what is a reasonable charge for these services.

Standard insurance coverage limits are usually defined by the following terms:

Medical Necessity — The service provided must be medically necessary. Services and tests that are not required will not be covered. As an example, sometimes the assistant surgeon's fees are denied because the procedure performed did not require an assistant surgeon. When this happens the patient will be responsible for the fee.

Accident or Illness — Most medical policies will cover only charges that resulted from an accident or an illness, therefore, charges for a well checkup are not covered, nor are birth control bills. Some of the newer policies that address preventative medicine now cover some of these services, but you must know your policy coverage.

UCR (Usual, Customary and Reasonable) — This is the way insurance companies limit the amount they will pay for services and is discussed in detail later in this chapter.

Experimental Treatments — Many insurance companies do not cover treatments that are not fully accepted by the medical community or for which the results of the treatment are ineffective. Many times new procedures are not covered until the risks and benefits of the treatment are proven. You should ask your physician if the treatment will be covered and if you will have to pay if it is not.

While insurance companies infrequently deny payment for all part of medical charges, they all have claim payment guidelines for medical procedures. Reasonable charge guidelines are an insurance company's only method of controlling fees charged for services. On a national basis, only 3 percent to 7 percent of all billings exceed usual, customary and reasonable charges.

Occasionally, you may receive a statement from the insurance company indicating that not all charges billed by the medical provider have been paid. Usually, this is accompanied with the phrase "charges exceed the usual, customary and reasonable charge (UCR)" or "inappropriate billing." This means that the insurance company has paid as much as the insurance contract will allow and the excess charges will be your responsibility.

Should this happen to you, you can review your billed charges and negotiate for relief of any excessive or inappropriate fees to reduce the financial hardship caused by the high fees. If you and the doctor have already previously agreed to waive excess fees as suggested in Chapter 6, "Ask Your Doctor," then the excessive charges shouldn't be a problem. Most of the time (90 percent), the negotiation will be successful and medical providers will waive these charges. If the physician will not waive the excess fees you may remind him of the AMA Ethics Standards which state "A fee is excessive when . . . a person knowledgeable as to current charges . . . would be left with a firm conviction that the fee is excessive." "A physician should not charge . . . or collect an excessive fee."

(NOTE: Excess charges *are not* your responsibility if you used a PPO provider. PPO provider contracts with insurance companies *do not* allow the physician to collect excess fees.)

HOW DOCTORS CHARGE

Doctors are reimbursed for services much like an automobile mechanic. When you have work performed on your car, the mechanic refers to a "flat rate" book which estimates how many hours it will take to fix the problem. He then bills his hourly rate times the estimated time given in the "flat rate" book.

The medical services industry also has a "flat rate" book with numerical codes (CPT codes) for medical procedures. Most of these codes are preprinted on doctors' billing forms. The doctor simply checks a box next to a procedure he performed and the office staff computes the charges.

Medical codes are assigned to each procedure according to its degree of difficulty. As an example, an office visit for an established patient has six different codes:

Sample Cost	CPT Code (Established Patient Visit)	Description	Services To Be Provided
$20	90030	Minimal Service	Injections, Dressings
$29	90040	Brief Examination	Minimal Physician Services
$43	90050	Limited Examination	Treatment and Discussion of Findings
$54	90060	Intermediate	Complete History, In-depth Counseling, Exam of One or More Organ Systems
$72	90070	Extended Reexamination	Service Requiring an Unusual Amount of Time
$108	90080	Comprehensive Reexamination	In-depth Patient Evaluation for an Unusually Complex Medical Problem

The cost shown will vary by location (less in Montana than Beverly Hills) and specialty. The cost of an office visit by a neurosurgeon will be more than an office visit by a family practice doctor.

****

CONCEPT AT WORK:

A Tale of Two Brothers — One brother and his wife went on vacation to Great Falls, Montana and the other brother stayed home. The spouse of the brother who went to Great Falls got sick and spent a full day in the hospital emergency room and had many diagnostic tests run to determine her illness. She was then admitted to the hospital for four more days. The total bill for all five days was $1,500.

The brother who stayed home took a daughter to the emergency room. Surgery was performed and the daughter returned home without a night in the hospital. The total bill for services was $4,300, $300 for the surgeon and $4,000 for the hospital.

The insurance company considered both hospital bills as reasonable charges.

****

If a physician submits a bill with fees higher than a majority of physicians in his area, the insurance company will exclude the excess and you will be responsible. When this happens the normal insurance company statement is "charges exceed UCR." In our example, if a physician billed $60 for CPT code 90060 (intermediate visit) and the UCR rate for that zip code was $40, the patient would be responsible for the excess charge of $20 ($60 - $40), the deductible and coinsurance.

Most insurance companies typically define "UCR" charges to cover 85 percent to 95 percent of the charges submitted in your zip code. This means that if a charge is defined a "excessive" it is a charge higher than 85 percent to 95 percent of the charges they have received for that procedure in your area.

The insurance company's method of defining "UCR" is probably one of the reasons for the high increase in medical cost. All doctors have to do is submit "excessive" charges one year and they become "normal" charges the following year because the insurance company's computer will recognize the many excessive charges and assume that is the normal rate for that zip code. Next year the "UCR" definition will change to cover 85 percent to 95 percent of the charges received and bingo, insurance rates go up.

Sometimes a provider will purposely file a high charge so that they can determine the maximum reimbursement from your insurance company. If enough providers file high charges they can increase the future definition of reasonable charges, as reasonable charges will then increase.

Sorry for the lengthy explanation of how doctors charge, but you can't be an active participant until you understand how the system works.

CREEPING CPT CODES

Patients may also become responsible for excess charges by physician manipulation of the CPT codes. There are a number of ways this can be done. The industry refers to this process as "creeping codes" since the cost of service creeps upwards when the codes are manipulated. All of these methods violate AMA Ethics Standards, as does the attempt to collect payment.

The four most common ways CPT codes can be manipulated to increase fees are

Unbundling
Exploding Tests
Changed Diagnosis
Upcoding

Unbundling

Unbundling occurs when a *single* medical procedure is separated into *numerous* procedures (steps) and then billed separately. The sum of the numerous individual procedures is generally many times more than the allowable cost for the single procedure.

Everyday Example		Medical Example	
Fix Flat Tire (normal charge)	$ 5	Hysterectomy (normal charge)	$2,500
Unbundled Charges:		Unbundled Charges:	
Jack-up Car	$ 5	Fallopian Tubes Removal	$2,000
Replace Tire	$ 5	Ovary Removal	$2,000
Fix Flat Tire	$ 5	Uterus Removal	$3,000
Wash Hands	N/C		
Charge	**$15**	**Charge**	**$7,000**
Additional You Pay	**$10**	**Additional You Pay**	**$4,500**

It is sometimes difficult for a patient to detect unbundling. If your insurance company rejects any charges as "inappropriate billing," it should be a red light that you could be the victim of unbundling.

When you buy unbundled medical services, it is like buying a new car part-by-part from the parts department at a cost of $80,000, rather than from the new car sales department for $15,000. Since we don't buy cars that way, why should we pay for unbundled medical services?

If the insurance company discovers this type of billing, it is obligated by AMA guidelines to pay at the rate of the single procedure code rather than the procedure codes for the steps.

****

CONCEPT AT WORK:

A young single parent making minimum wage had surgery for which the doctor billed $4,500 and the insurance company considered $2,500 as "reasonable." The parent was treated very nicely by the doctor and was allowed to set up a payment schedule of $30 a month for five years. Later the patient complained to the employer about the "lousy" benefits and insurance company. The employer looked at the claim and suspected unbundling. The concept was discussed with the parent. The parent took these suspicions to the doctor and the charges were waived. She no longer had the financial hardship of a $30 a month payment for five years.

****

Exploding Tests

"Exploding tests" apply to lab work. The process is similar to the "unbundling" of medical procedures. Several tests from several samples are charged although one combined test from a single sample could provide the same results.

Normal Test	Charge
Chemical Profile (SMAC) (A Blood Chemistry Test)	$ 30
Separate Test for	
Cholesterol	20
Glucose	20
Hemoglobin	30
Red Blood Cell Count	30
White Blood Cell Count	20
Uric Acid	26
EXPLODED TEST CHARGE	**$145**
YOU PAY	**$115**

The one SMAC blood chemistry test can test and report the same results as the *seven* separate tests. Most blood tests are now done mechanically and most of the test cost is for the lab to handle the sample, not the actual testing process.

Again, the insurance company will only pay for the cost of the combined test, rather than the cost of the individual tests.

Changed Diagnosis

"Changed diagnosis" occurs when a bill is submitted for one diagnosis and the doctor's notes indicate a different diagnosis for the purpose of ensuring payment by the insurance company. This may happen when we have a routine physical, which is not commonly covered by medical plans, and the doctor codes a diagnosis (*i.e.,* heart palpitations) that can be covered by the insurance plan.

Upcoding

"Upcoding" is a method in which the service provided differs from the service billed. An example is if a patient had a 2 cm wound repaired and the doctor billed services to repair a 10 cm wound. If the difference between services "billed" and "provided" is caught by the insurance company from the doctor's notes, it will only pay for the 2 cm wound repair, which is the actual service provided. It is your responsibility to be sure that billed services are the same as performed services, since you might be liable for the difference.

While "upcoding" of some services may be difficult for the consumer to recognize, the consumer can *easily* recognize the most frequent abuse of "upcoding," *the office visit.* Many times a brief office visit (90040) is upcoded to a limited examination (90050) or intermediate (90060). Many doctors don't even have a minimal services (90030) listed on their preprinted bills.

One insurance company in one city analyzed 80,000 office visits over a 6 month period. The percentage of visits were: minimal services — 2 percent, brief — 8 percent, limited — 43 percent, intermediate — 42 percent, extended — 2 percent, and comprehensive — 3 percent. If all visits were upcoded only one step the cost difference would be $2 million a year. Two million dollars a year for one insurance company in one city extended to just 10 insurance companies in 10 cities would be $200 million and *only the consumer knows if upcoding occurred.*

Medicare has recognized the problem of upcoding office visits and is trying to implement a new method of paying for office visits based on time spent with the patient. The current plan is to start this new system January 1, 1992 and phase in over a five year period.

	Old Method	New Method	
Code	Description	Time	% Billed
90030	Minimal Service	5 Minutes	2%
90040	Brief Examination	10 Minutes	8%
90050	Limited Examination	15 Minutes	43%
90060	Intermediate	20 Minutes	42%
90070	Extended Reexamination	30 Minutes	2%
90080	Comprehensive Reexamination	60 Minutes	3%

We provide this table so the consumer can better judge the service provided. Using time to measure service will help control the most commonly abused "upcoding."

How prevalent is upcoding?   Very prevalent, if studies and consumer experience show physicians spend only 7 to 11 minutes (specialists spend more time, neurosurgeons spend 24 minutes) with the patient and 85 percent of the billings are services of 15 to 20 minutes. Think of all your visits, how many were less than 10 minutes and how many times did you spend 15 to 20 minutes with the physician?

The next time you visit the doctor, check the time spent.

All four of these methods of CPT code manipulation increase the cost of your medical care, but do not necessarily increase the quality of your care.   The examples shown are illustrative only. Actual cost differences for treatment can amount to $5,000, $10,000 or more, so you have to be careful. Some insurance companies may catch these "creeping codes" and deny the excessive charges as "exceeding the usual, reasonable and customary charges" or "inappropriate billing." Most likely, the medical provider will look to you for payment unless you have predetermined that your doctor will waive the excessive charges or you discuss the violation of AMA Ethics Standards.

What Can You Do?

When you receive your notice that the insurance company has paid the healthcare provider and find that you owe more than the deductible and co-insurance amounts, take these steps:

Step 1 - Check to see if charges were not paid because services were not covered by your policy.

Action: Not much you can do but appeal to insurance company to pay or ask provider to waive or reduce charges. You should ask the insurance company to give you the page number and clause of their contract which excluded coverage. Sometimes this will allow you to provide a better explanation of why you think it should be covered.

Step 2 - Check to see if healthcare provider was a PPO member. If they are a PPO provider, by contract they cannot collect the excessive fee amount from the patient.

Action: Note such on insurance work sheet and return to provider. Many times services such as labs, radiology, pathology, etc. perform work at the direction of your doctor. If your PPO doctor requested services of a non-PPO provider after you expressed a desire for only PPO providers, then the discussion of excessive charges should be referred to your doctor because you did not authorize their services nor did you have a choice. Simply state so on the bill and refer them to your doctor. It is not your problem, your wishes were not followed.

Step 3 - Check to see if the insurance company considered the charges as "excessive" or "unreasonable."

Action: Send a copy of the letter shown below quoting AMA ethics.

Step 4 - Check to see if insurance company considered charges "inappropriate." "Inappropriate" charges usually mean charges submitted by healthcare providers resulted from creeping codes.

Action: Indicate to provider that you feel Billing Department made a coding mistake and ask for charges to be waived. You may also appeal to the local medical boards/societies, and as a last resort, you may consider fraud charges.

Filing fraud charges may seem drastic, but "creeping codes" are wrong and costly without any benefit to the patient. The General Accounting Office (GAO) reported that 20 percent of the Medicare claims were inaccurate at a cost of $300 plus million.

If the insurance company denies payment of a portion of the provider's charges due to "excessive charges" or "inappropriate billing," you may try sending a letter such as this.

Dear Dr. _____:

I have received my insurance company's explanation of benefits (attached) for services provided by you.

Please notice their reduction of your charges as noted by the statement "Charges exceed the prevailing rate for this geographic area." If you feel that you have miscoded your services rendered, please correct and resubmit to the insurance company.

If you feel that your services are coded correctly, I would like you to waive these "excessive charges" as per the American Medical Association *Current Opinions of the Council of Ethical and Judicial Affairs Section 6.12* (copy attached) which states:

> A physician should not charge or collect an illegal or excessive fee. . . . A fee is excessive when after review of the facts a person knowledgeable as to the current charges made by physicians would be left with a definite and firm conviction that the fee is in excess of a reasonable fee. . . .

It is my opinion that an insurance company's claims payer is "a person knowledgeable as to current charges." Insurance companies pay 80% of the charges billed by medical providers and I believe this qualifies them as "a knowledgeable person."

As you are aware, the *Current Opinions* are intended "standards of conduct which define essentials of honorable behavior for the physician." I presume that the charges will be waived unless I hear further from you.

Sincerely,

Patient

You should modify this sample letter to your particular situation and use the wording on the insurance company work sheet.

WHEN INSURANCE COMPANIES PAY TOO MUCH

Most healthcare providers are very honest, hardworking and ethical. Occasionally, however, you might encounter situations in which you suspect the physician, lab or hospital has charged too much. As the consumer, you have the right to be fully informed about your healthcare costs. You, the consumer, should be on the lookout for misleading marketing gimmicks, such as "free services" or "increased services."

Free Services

Some medical providers now advertise "free services" to attract patients. Often this means services are "free" to you and you will not have to pay your deductible or coinsurance payment. The insurance company, however, may be charged for tests, services and treatments not performed or the charges for services may be excessive. Total charges billed to the insurance company may be three, four, even ten times higher than services provided.

Do not be misled by "free services." Ask to see the charges to be billed to your insurance company. If you didn't receive the tests or the charges are high, protest them with the provider and the insurance company. If you visit a free service provider, compare the charges, diagnosis and treatment with another provider before entering treatment. We all know that free services or items are provided as an inducement to increase business revenue. Why should it be any different in the medical services industry?

****

CONCEPT AT WORK:

How Much Do "Free Services" Cost? One insurance company recently received an $18 million award from a lab that was submitting claims for services not rendered, but for which claims were filed and paid by the insurance company. Until the insurance company receives their $18 million, the employers and employees in that area will have to pay higher insurance rates.

****

Increased Services

Insurance companies that have installed PPO programs have noticed that claims cost have not decreased, despite the fact that the insurance company has negotiated substantial discounts for medical services.

The insurance companies have found that, while the unit cost of service is lower (because of tough provider negotiations), the number of visits for service or the amount of service provided has increased resulting in increased claims cost, rather than a decrease.

An actual example of this occurred when a patient received treatment on a quarterly basis. The regular charge was $85 which the patient paid. With a switch in the patient's employer paid insurance coverage to a PPO program, the doctor stated the employee no longer needed to pay his portion and the doctor would bill the insurance company directly. The patient's next visit cost the insurance company $285 for the same services which had previously cost the patient $85. The physician simply billed the insurance company for more services, while providing the patient with the same treatment.

If this happens to you, bring it to your doctor's attention and ask your insurance company for assistance. The insurance company will need a copy of your old bill and the new bill to determine how the charges were manipulated and probably, in addition, a statement from you. If this is too difficult for you, you may want to consider switching doctors. If the doctor cheats on the bill, what else may he be doing?

Some insurance companies now aggressively pursue healthcare providers who file fraudulent claims. If you feel your provider has fraudulently filed claims you may contact the insurance company and file a complaint with your state Attorney General.

PLEASE REMEMBER THAT ANY CHARGE THE INSURANCE COMPANY PAYS THIS YEAR, YOU WILL PAY NEXT YEAR IN INCREASED PREMIUMS.

SUMMARY

Many of us feel we have adequate medical insurance. In reality, there is no such thing as insurance, it is simply a delayed billing system. You have seen this delayed billing concept illustrated by insurance rate adjustments occurring every year for the last ten years. Rate adjustments are supported when medical claims exceed medical premiums. In reality, our medical insurance system is merely a medical charge system. **WHATEVER WE CHARGE THIS YEAR WILL HAVE TO BE PAID NEXT YEAR PLUS THE MEDICAL INFLATION RATE OF 20 PERCENT TO 30 PERCENT.**

It is in our best interest therefore to shop for medical services as if we were *purchasing* medical services, rather than simply consuming them.

Use your medical benefits I.D. card like a charge card and shop carefully. Ask questions, compare prices, check references and thoroughly discuss your treatment plan with your medical provider. REMEMBER, YOU WILL HAVE TO PAY FOR IT NEXT YEAR.

The Most Expensive

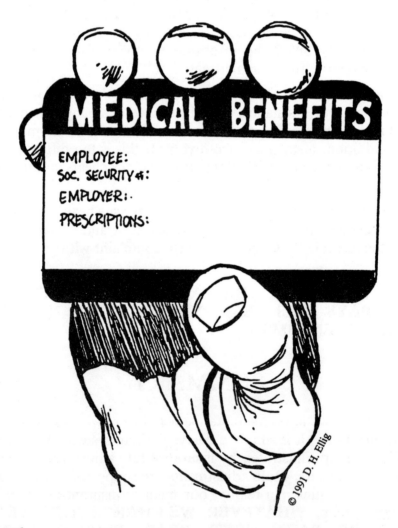

Charge Card In Your Wallet!

CHAPTER 16

MENTAL HEALTHCARE

Mental healthcare cost is the fastest growing area of employer benefit plans, with some employers experiencing increases of 50 percent yearly. The following increase illustrates this rapid growth: billings from psychiatric specialty hospitals have increased seven times in only seven years ($2 billion in 1982 to $14 billion in 1989).

Mental healthcare is the one medical service area in which the consumer is subjected to advertising. Unfortunately, advertising is sponsored by the most costly treatment facilities — in–hospital treatment. Consumers view ads on TV, billboards, newspapers and radio. Advertising messages effectively suggest you or a loved one might be in need of help and these facilities are there to help (and everyone will live happily ever after). Fortunately, only a small portion of the population suffers from a mental illness requiring hospitalization. Yet it is the treatment plan which is most often presented to us via the advertising media. (Obviously it is effective if hospital billings have increased seven times.)

INTRODUCTION

For the consumer, mental healthcare can also be the most confusing area for treatment. Most of us are mentally healthy but must deal with the ordinary problems of living. When we seek help from mental healthcare providers, we are usually in the "worried well" category which responds to outpatient treatment visits. "Worried well" are those people who suffer from lifestyle stresses and need only mental health wellness checkups and assurances. Sometimes we just need to be reassured that we can work our problems out and get on with our lives. We are not alone, we just need a little professional guidance.

Most "worried well" patients usually respond to one to six outpatient provider visits, depending on the extent of the illness. It is becoming more and more socially acceptable for people to admit to being a "worried well" person and seek a few outpatient treatments. Most people do not require hospitalization. They function well in society after only a few outpatient treatments. National figures show that 77 percent of patients respond to outpatient treatment, 18 percent to partial hospitalization and only 5 percent require inpatient hospitalization.

For the lay person entering the mental health system it can be very confusing because there are many different types of illnesses, providers, qualifications and accreditations.

LICENSING PROVIDERS

As an example, most states do not credential or license the majority of mental health providers. Many states license only psychiatrists (M.D. or D.O.). However, most states are now credentialing a variety of mental health providers in their area of expertise. In addition, some providers are accredited by professional organizations.

The words licensing, credentialing and accredited are important and should be understood.

Licensing is normally done by the state and means that a provider cannot practice without a state license. It is mandatory that the provider have a license.

Credentialing is also normally done by the state but is a voluntary process. The provider must apply to be credentialed, but can practice without being credentialed. The credentialing process normally involves the state reviewing the provider's educational background, work experience, and passing grade on a state sponsored test.

Accreditation is normally provided by a professional organization and is also voluntary.

DIFFERENT PROVIDERS

Mental healthcare services can be provided by many different degree-qualified providers. A sample list is shown on on the following page:

Psychiatrist (M.D.) — only provider who can prescribe drugs as part of
   treatment plan
Clinical Psychologist (Ph.D.)
Master Degreed (M.S. or M.A.)
   Marriage and Family Therapist
   Social Worker (M.S.W.)
   Counselors (M.C.)

---

*The above providers normally practice without supervision. The providers
below normally provide services only under the supervision of one of the above
or in an agency.*

*Bachelor level providers normally do not provide unsupervised services directly
to patients in an outpatient setting.*

Bachelor of Science Degreed (B.S. or B.A.)
   Marriage and Family Therapist
   Social Worker (B.S.W.)
   Counselors
Clinical Psychiatric Registered Nurses (R.N.)
Non-Degreed
   Addiction Counselors

The cost of these providers will vary. Generally the psychiatrist is the most
expensive and the nondegreed is the least expensive. Among the various providers,
an additional cost factor would be whether the provider is licensed, credentialed
or accredited.

Selecting a mental health provider can be difficult. It is therefore, best to get
references. Here are several ways to obtain provider references:

Community referral systems/crisis hotlines/support groups
References from clergy, teachers, physicians, lawyers
Your employer's Employee Assistance Program (EAP)
A local EAP firm
Another mental healthcare provider who specializes in your area of treatment
A referral from a friend who has been treated for a similar problem

Mental health providers specialize in certain mental illness conditions just as
medical doctors do. Nevertheless, you may want to enter the system through a
mental health counselor, since your condition may be caused by several

overlapping problems. It is quite common to have a primary diagnosis and several secondary diagnoses.

The mental health counselor can define the primary diagnosis, if necessary, and refer you to a provider who specializes in your problem. The mental health counselor may refer you to a medical doctor if it is suspected your condition may result from a medical problem. You should, however, be prepared to pay for the initial consulting interview.

Some conditions that mental health providers treat are listed below:

Addiction	Marriage/Family Problems	Life Transitions
Alcohol	Anxiety/Depression	Adolescence Crises
Drugs	Suicidal Problems	Middle Life Crises
Sex	Grief	Aging Anxieties
Food	Stress	Death and Dying Crises
Gambling	Obsessive Compulsive Disorders	
Codependency		

If you need a specialist, the next step is to interview the selected provider for qualifications. You might have to pay for an initial provider qualification interview, although you might be able to get most of your answers from his staff.

PROVIDER QUALIFYING

Once you have selected your providers for the interview, you need to ask some questions.

It is important to use some tact when asking these questions in order not to offend the provider. Explain that you don't know who they are or their qualifications. Most providers will be happy to tell you how good they are if you give them the chance and ask the questions in a nonconfrontational manner.

* Are you a preferred provider (PPO) for my employer's benefit plan?

* What is your degree qualification?

* How long have you been treating *this specific condition*?

It is hoped that by now you know your specific condition from discussions with a generalist. If not, you may have to extend your interview process to include a mental health wellness checkup.

* Are you licensed, credentialed, or accredited?

    Examples are:

    > American Board of Psychiatric in Child Psychology
    > American Board of Psychiatry and Neurology
    > Academy of Certified Social Workers (A.C.S.W.)
    > Certified Marriage and Family Therapists
    > Certified Counselor
    > Certified Addiction Professional (C.A.P.)
    > Certified Alcohol Counselor
    > Certified Drug Counselor
    > Certified Alcohol and Drug Abuse Counselor
    > Accredited in Adolescent Psychology
    > Certified Clinical Psychologist
    > Certified Counseling Psychologist

* Are you licensed to practice in this area? (Some states do not require licensing or accreditation.)

* What percentage of your patients treated for my condition do you refer to inpatient programs? (3 percent is average, higher for addictions.)

* What is your criteria for referring patients to inpatient treatment facilities?

    Most admissions to inpatient treatment programs can only be made by M.D.s or D.O.s.

* Which facility do you refer to and why?

* How long is your average treatment plan? (Average is 3 to 12 visits, more for addictive disorders.)

* Will the treatment plan include the individual only or will all family members be included?

    Many treatment programs now suggest that the entire family group receive counseling. This helps the professional with problem definition and also helps family members understand the problem so that they may become part of the treatment plan.

* How often will we meet?

    Most often a treatment plan will require frequent meetings at the beginning, tapering off as progress is made.

* Will you provide a list of support groups?

Support groups provide a very important source to other people who have experienced or are experiencing your problem. The sharing of experiences will help both the patient and family members.

* Do you recommend attendance at support group meetings?

* What is your hourly fee? Do you have a sliding scale or prepaid treatment package?

* Can I schedule my sessions during nonworking hours?

* If you are seeking treatment for addiction ask: Are you, yourself, a recovering *(fill-in the blank)?* How long?

You should pick a qualified provider with whom you feel comfortable. It is extremely important that you are comfortable with your therapist or counselor/client relationship, because it will normally provide quicker and better results.

OUTPATIENT VERSUS IN-HOSPITAL COSTS

Mental health services are provided at a variety of locations:

a) Outpatient office visits (1 hour sessions, the famous 50-minute hour)

b) Intensive outpatient treatment (3 to 4 hour sessions, 5 days)

c) Partial hospitalization (day hospitalization — 8 hour days)

d) Residential treatment programs (hospitalization for X days)

e) Inpatient acute care facilities (hospitalization for X days)

The costs for these treatment programs vary considerably. To the consumer, this will be a very important consideration, since most employer benefit plans have separate coinsurance schedules and plan maximums for mental health. As such, it is possible that the consumer's share of a mental illness treatment program's cost can be more expensive than traditional medical treatment plans. For example, many benefit programs only pay 50 percent of the mental healthcare cost versus the traditional 80 or 100 percent coverage for a medical provider. Also, it is not uncommon for outpatient mental illness visits to be limited to $1,000 yearly, with a $10,000 to $100,000 lifetime maximum payment for inpatient treatment. Estimates of 1991 costs are as follows:

a) Outpatient office visits $40/$120 hour

b) Intensive outpatient treatment $90/$200 day

c) Partial hospitalization $100/$300 day

d) Residential treatment programs $130/$400 day

e) Inpatient acute care facilities $300/$1,000 plus day

Costs will vary according to the provider qualifications previously discussed, such as licensing, credentialing, and accreditation. Normally the more licensing, credentialing, and accreditation the provider has, the higher the provider billing rate.

IN-HOSPITAL TREATMENT

If it is determined from discussions with the mental health counselor or the lack of progress by the outpatient treatment plan that hospitalization is required, the following section will assist you to qualify a facility. Most in-hospital treatments are designed for addictive illnesses, adolescent treatment, and the severely ill who may be a threat to themselves or others.

You should carefully consider the need for in-hospital treatment plans, since there is much debate among mental health providers regarding the effectiveness of in-hospital treatment versus outpatient treatment. This debate is illustrated in a recent University of Michigan study of 20,000 hospitalized adolescents. The study found that 75 percent of the adolescent hospitalizations were inappropriate or potentially harmful to the child or family over the long run and, with the exception of extreme cases, were no more effective than outpatient treatment programs.

Adolescent hospital admissions have increased dramatically in the last 20 years and show the following growth:

                    1970 — 7,000
                    1980 — 13,000
                    1990 —150,000 (estimated)

The explosive growth in adolescent hospital admissions could be due to increased advertising, combined with the public's lack of knowledge about other treatment programs and increased lifestyle pressures faced by teenagers.

It is extremely important that once you decide inpatient treatment is necessary, you carefully qualify the facility, because of the high cost ($1,000 plus a day) and length of treatment plans (30, 60, 90 days and longer). In-hospital treatment plans are a large part of the cost increase in employer health plans, as cost of treatment can range from $20,000 to $100,000.

Inpatient hospitalization is readily available because of the large increase in hospital beds. The number of private beds has almost doubled (83 percent increase in the last five years, 1983 to 1989). The possibility exists that if you or a loved one present yourself at an inpatient facility, you will be admitted, even if the diagnosis does not indicate hospitalization is necessary or hospital treatment is appropriate.   Many employer programs now require precertification of in-hospital mental illness admissions. This is a result of rapidly increasing cost and occasional inappropriate admissions.

Although inpatient mental healthcare is extremely expensive, most people place high value on the prospect of a loved one functioning normally. To most people, treatment is worth $70,000, $80,000, $120,000, particularly if an insurance company will pay. Not many can afford inpatient treatment without insurance and have to find another treatment plan or rely on public funding.

Once you are sure that hospitalization is required, the following discussion will help you select the appropriate facility:

FACILITY QUALIFYING

Qualification Questions For

Partial Hospitalization (Day Care)
Residential Treatment Programs
Inpatient Acute Care

* Did you call your insurance company to precertify your hospital stay? If not, you may have to pay a larger share of the cost of treatment.

* If your program has preferred providers (PPO), do you know if all of the professionals providing services are PPO providers?

    Many medical plans have different payment schedules for PPO providers and non-PPO providers. If you use non-PPO providers, your cost for medical services will increase. Therefore, it would be beneficial to assure that hospital, labs and *all* doctors who provide services are PPO providers.

    If some of the providers are non-PPO providers, you may want to discuss this with your primary physician and consider asking the non-PPO providers to waive fees not covered by the insurance company.

* Must a doctor (M.D.) admit you to facility?

* What is the professional staff (counselors) to patient ratio? (A ratio of greater than 1 to 8 is too high, a ratio of 1 to 6 is better, with the exception of adolescent treatment, in which a ratio of 1 to 2 or 1 to 1 is best.)

* Does the facility use master level and Ph.D. candidate students for direct counseling? Does it employ students who are in training for B.S. or B.A. degrees?

    What services do students provide? At what charge?

Will they be identified as students?

* Ask for a list of staff members showing credentials, degrees, specialties and accreditation.

* Ask how long each staff member has been at the facility. (The longer the treatment team has worked together, the greater the possibility that you're working with a stable organization.)

* What is the staff turnover rate?

* Does the facility provide treatment goals, a timetable of achieving those goals, and a measurement program of daily progress to reach those goals?

This is an extremely important question. You should compare the treatment plan length to your benefit coverage as most treatment plans will cease when benefits are exhausted. If the treatment length or cost exceeds your benefits, you may want to discuss alternatives now, rather than when benefits are exhausted.

* If admitting for addiction, what is the percentage of recovering counselors, for how long, and what type of training do the counselors have?

There is some dispute among mental care providers concerning the use of recovered addictive personalities as counselors. Those in support say it is best because the recovered addict has experienced the addiction and can communicate effectively with the patient because of shared experiences. Those against use of recovered addictive counselors say they are not required to have "professional" training and that they have too much empathy which causes them to be too easy on the patient.

* What treatment model does your facility use?

There are two broad treatment models used to treat addictive illness: behavioral and spirituality. The AA 12-Step Program has some spirituality aspects that a nonspiritual patient may have some difficulty accepting. Treatment may therefore be difficult.

* What type of outpatient follow-up service does the facility provide and at what cost?

What type of relapse program is available?

Is the relapse program fee included?

* What are the daily fees?

* What do the fees cover?

Are the professional fees included in the facility fees?

Are psychological testing fees included in the facility fees?

Are medical testing fees included in the facility fees?

* Do the fees include family therapy while the patient is in treatment and after release and for how long?

* How many counseling hours will be provided daily? How many hours will be individual counseling? How many hours will be group therapy? Will there be counseling in the evenings and on weekends?

* If admitted on a weekend, when will treatment begin?
  (In many facilities treatment for new admittees is not available over the weekend.)

* What restrictions will be placed on individuals during treatment? What about home passes?

   If the treatment plan is progressing well enough for the individual to have home passes and outside privileges, you should seriously discuss the need for continued in-hospital treatment and the possibility of a switch to intensive outpatient treatment.

* Will telephone privileges be allowed? Outgoing only or outgoing and incoming?

* For adolescent treatment ask these questions:

   Does the facility have a "lockup" area to prevent patient runaways?

   What ages are admitted and is there age and sex separation?

   How will school work be continued and transferred?

* Are support group meetings offered at the facility? How often?

* Is the facility accredited by the Joint Commission on the Accreditation of Health Care Organizations (JCAHO)?

   Almost all facilities will be accredited by JCAHO, since it qualifies the facility for payment of government funds.

* Is the facility accredited by the Commission on Accreditation of Rehabilitation Facilities (CARF)?

   This accreditation is often associated with facilities that specialize in substance abuse treatment programs.

SUPPORT GROUPS

It is extremely important that the individual seeking treatment and family members be aware of the availability of support group organizations. Many times we think we are the only ones with this condition or experience. Support groups are extremely helpful since members have been through the same problem and can share their experiences. We suggest you check locally and ask the hospital for support groups.

Also refer to our chapter on Support Groups for toll-free phone numbers.

MENTAL HEALTH SELF-HELP BOOKS

Below are some readings which may be beneficial to the individual and the family.

A word of warning. These are popular books and may not be available when you visit the library. As an example, a recent visit to the library found that of the 24 books referenced 14 were on loan, 5 were lost and only 5 were available. It may be best to visit your local book store.

Substance Abuse:

Goodbye Hangovers, Hello Life and Turnabout, by Jean Kirkpatric

A self-help book for women addressing the special needs of women alcoholics. Written by a former alcoholic, it discusses the "new life" program and principles of women for sobriety. Deals with the negative emotions that make it difficult for the drinking alcoholic to recover; worry, fear, guilt, depression and loneliness.

Not My Kid, by Beth Polson and Miller Newton

This book is written by a clinical drug therapist and discusses drug problems and practical solutions for families with children with drug problems.

Discusses tools to insure that drugs don't invade the house, early warning signs of drug use and where to turn for assistance when a drug problem is discovered.

The 100 Best Treatment Centers for Alcohol and Drug Abuse, by Sunshine and Wright, Avon Books

This book is the result of a survey of drug and alcohol abuse professionals. One hundred treatment facilities are listed, with descriptions of treatment programs, costs, and locations.

The survey questions used to select and evaluate the facilities are also provided. These questions may be helpful to those individuals who wish to evaluate a facility not listed. Be aware that some of the data may change since the book was written in 1988 and the survey completed previously.

Sitting in the Baywindow: A Book For Parents of Young Alcoholics, by Jack Mumey

This book offers advice to parents suffering with teenage drinking problems. Provides solutions on how to handle the various situations which occur and addresses the parental guilt feelings.

Discusses the various types of treatment programs available and what your expectations should be.

Depression:

Depression and Its Treatment: Help for the Nation's #1 Mental Problem, by John H. Greist, M.D., and James W. Jefferson, M.D.

This is a small book written by two professors of psychiatry and is very simple to understand. It discusses what depression is, how it's treated, treatment side effects and how to interact with your doctor.

Feeling Good: The New Mood Therapy, by David D. Burns

Outlines a systematic program for controlling thought disorders that lead to low esteem and depression. It discusses how we can alter our moods to deal with emotional problems by changing the way we think. Discusses how childhood patterns of relating are continued in adult relationships and how they may be changed.

Is Your Child Depressed?, by Joel Herskowitz, M.D.

Unlike adults, depressed children may not appear sad or depressed, just off in their normal behavior patterns. This book is written by a pediatric neurologist and discusses how to recognize depression in children and how to help. It provides step-by-step guidelines and checklists to recognize depression. It also prepares parents for mental health counseling if it is needed by describing treatment patterns and medications. It discusses the causes and prevention of suicides.

Codependency:

Codependent No More, How to Stop Controlling Others and Start Caring for Yourself, by Melody Beattie

Written by a recovering alcoholic and former dependent counselor, this book discusses codependency, how it affects us, where it comes from, what it is and several options for changing behavior. It discusses how people take so much responsibility for those that are not taking responsibility that it affects the person without the problem.

The author also has a second book *Beyond Codependency* that expands the ideas developed in *Codependent No More*.

Do I Have to Give Up Me to be Loved By You?, by Jordan and Margaret Paul

This book about marital relationships is written by a husband and wife team of psychologists. The book explores why couples behave as they do, how relationships get into trouble and to handle conflict. The theory presented is that most of our couple behavioral actions are motivated by self-protection from the other party's disapproval and fear of rejection.

Exercises are provided to explore your true feelings, thoughts and provide help to change your way of handling conflicts.

Men Who Hate Women and the Women Who Love Them, by Dr. Susan Forward

A book about women in a relationship with emotionally abusive men. Discusses how some men can love a woman and yet cause them pain by their actions and words. An emotionally abusive relationship can be very destructive to a woman's self-esteem. However, the book provides guidance on how to understand, handle and recover, either by rebuilding the relationship or getting out.

Women Who Love Too Much, by Robin Norwood

This book addresses how some women are drawn into unhappy and destructive relationships with men and then attempt to make the relationship work.

Life Transitions:

Children of Alcoholics, by Robert Ackerman, Ph.D.

The book describes how to help and find help for children in alcoholic families. The book discusses how to recognize alcoholism and how to cope with children's behavioral problems. The book gives some ideas on how children can cope with the alcoholic family situation.

Cutting Loose, by Howard Halpern

Halpern discusses how adults can be stuck with frustrating parent/child patterns even as adults. Even as adults we may continue to act as children in our relationship with our adult parents. The book provides ideas/methods to break the child/parent relationship and to replace it with adult/adult relationships.

The 40 to 60 Year Old Male, by Michael E. McGill

This book is subtitled, "A Guide for Men and the Women in Their Lives to See Them Through the Crisis of the Male Middle Years." Research for the book included interviews with approximately 250 men and their wives, children and associates. It discusses the difference between childhood goals and actual midlife achievement or lack thereof.

Making Peace With Your Parents, by Harold Bloomfield, M.D.

This book is written by a practicing psychiatrist as a result of his own personal experience with his mother and father. Bloomfield discusses the problem many of us have expressing our love and anger toward our parents. It provides exercises to break away from the approval trap and to deal with our parents aging, dying and death.

It is an extremely important book since all of us have a deep desire to love and be loved by our parents, but have a difficult time expressing, communicating and making the initial steps to open up the dialogue and feelings.

What Color is Your Parachute, by Richard Nelson Bolles

This cheery book for those in a career-changing job hunt, provides ideas for life and work planning in a light tone. First published in 1972, it has been updated annually with a full reference section.

Marriage and Family:

Back from Betrayal — Recovering from His Affair, by Jennifer P. Schneider, M.D.

This book is written by a physician who is the wife of a recovering sex addict. It is based on their personal experiences and outlines paths to recoveries with suggested steps that are illustrated from actual case examples. The recovery program uses the concepts of the 12-step program and suggests guidelines for choosing a counselor.

Elements of codependency and addiction counseling are mentioned frequently and used. The book is written for both women who decide to remain in the relationship and those who decide to terminate the relationship.

The Mirages of Marriage, by William Lederer and Dr. Don Jackson

This book discusses the complexities of marriage. It addresses some of the false assumptions of modern marriage and shows how to make a marriage work by providing an outline for a satisfactory marriage.

Parent Power, by John K. Rosemond

Written by a practicing child psychologist, this book covers the parents role in raising children from birth through the teenage years. It discusses children's growth stages and the problems they may present to parents. The book contains many situations, often humorous, and offers advice for handling problems.

Tough Love, by Phyllis and David York

Tough Love is a loving solution for parents whose teenagers have unacceptable behavior. It is written by the co-founders of the Tough Love program. The book discusses how parents can form their own support group to share the acting out experiences of their children. It shows how anticipation and preparation for a teenager's crisis can lead to positive change. The Yorks have also written another book *Tough Love Solutions.*

Others:

6,892 Questionable Doctors - Disciplined by States or the Federal Government, Published by a public citizen health research group report, June 1990

This book lists, by state, doctors who have had some type of action filed and were disciplined for various charges by both state and federal government agencies.

It is a good book to refer to, particularly if you are new in an area. The book provider certain qualifications and suggested cautions on its use. The book is available at public libraries in the reference section and some libraries will provide a service of researching the doctors name over the telephone.

The Courage to Heal — A Guide to Women Survivors of Child and Sexual Abuse, by Ellen Bass and Laura Davis

This book is cowritten by a survivor of child sexual abuse and her counselor. It covers the various healing processes, self-awareness, how to change, references to support groups, self-help programs and organizations.

Lonely All the Time, by Dr. Ralph Earle and Dr. Gregory Crow
(Recognizing, Understanding and Overcoming Sex Addiction for Addicts and Co-Dependents)

This is a fairly recent book about sex addiction, it discusses what it is, how it affects the family and how to recover. The book will help you understand what is sex addiction, how it can affect the family and how family members can recognize it and cope with it. Book covers sex addiction in its many forms, multiple affairs, pornography, prostitution services, exhibitionists, voyeurs and others. Finally the book presents a program for recovering from the addiction.

Out of the Shadows — Understanding Sexual Addiction, by Patrick Carnes

The book is written by one of the pioneers in the field of sexual addiction and discusses a 12-step program, plus the help of support groups as a treatment method. It indicates that sexual compulsiveness is an addiction, which causes shame, fear of abandonment, plus the feeling of aloneness in this addiction. The book discusses cases, treatments and successes.

Psycho-Cybernetics, by Maxwell Maltz, M.D.

This book was written by a plastic surgeon who discovered that patients still considered themselves disfigured even after he had changed disfiguring characteristics. It discusses how the mind can influence a person's perception of oneself and how one can use the mind to improve self-image.

When I Say No, I Feel Guilty, by Manuel Smith

This book was first published in 1975 and continues to be an excellent source of ideas for those who are constantly over-committing ourselves to projects, committees, tasks and activities that we don't really want to do. The book provides training exercises to help you say no without feeling guilty or losing your temper. This was one of the first books on assertive training.

And finally a book that provides an excellent reference source to more readings.

Consumer Health Information Source Book, by Alan M. Rees and Catherine Hoffman

This book provides an excellent source of published material in healthcare for the medical consumer. It contains book reviews on 750 books, 75 medical newsletters and 700 pamphlets. A quick reference to this book will give you direction to many excellent detailed sources.

NOTES

"Not Me" Circle

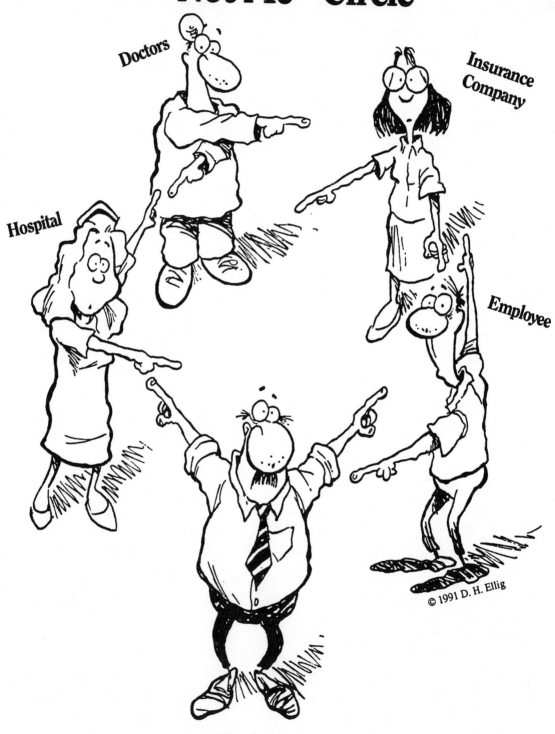

Doctors

Insurance Company

Hospital

Employee

Employer

© 1991 D. H. Ellig

CHAPTER 17

WHY HEALTHCARE IS *SO* EXPENSIVE

Healthcare services consumed 12 percent of the United States gross national product (GNP) in 1990, with military expenses not much higher. Employer provided medical benefits can consume as much as 50 percent of an employer's profits, which is money the corporation can't put into retirement plans, salaries, etc. The HEALTHCARE SERVICE INDUSTRY IS BIG BUSINESS. While the healthcare industry is BIG BUSINESS, access to it is controlled by only .2 percent (two tenths) of the United States population (500,000 doctors). Twelve percent of the GNP is controlled by 500,000 small businesses that gross $250,000 to over $1,000,000 a year with pre-tax profit margins of 60 percent.

What is amazing is that most people don't think of healthcare as a business, sometimes even the people running the business don't think of it as a business. No *real business* would dare treat their customers like patients are treated. No other customer would wait 45 minutes for services and then accept rude treatment when they ask about prices or quality of care.

That medical services is a **business** is one of the unique features of the United States healthcare delivery system. In most other industrialized countries healthcare is a **government** function and as such regulated and controlled by the government. Supplying healthcare service in the United States costs more than in all the other industrialized nations. Why is that? Could it be that the United States healthcare business has marketing features which are unique and not available to any other industry in the United States? The medical services industry operates like no other business in the United States.

The unique features of the United States healthcare industry lead to:

— **Lack of responsibility for costs**
— **Supply/demand players confusing**
— **Healthcare providers playing by different rules**
— **Lack of quality definition**

Nearly everyone in the United States is affected by the medical services industry. Most of us have had some experience with medical services, either for oneself, a child, or an aging parent.

Medical services have become very expensive for the ordinary individual. For the self-employed or the individual whose employer does not provide medical insurance, medical services are often unaffordable. It is not uncommon for the cost of medical insurance for a family of four to equal the cost of a house or car payment. Most families would rather have a home or a car than health insurance. The high cost of healthcare services leads to more uninsured patients, which ultimately creates more strain on the payer of medical services — you — through taxes, health premiums, deductibles and coinsurance. Our uninsured population is increasing daily and is currently estimated at 37,000,000.

NO ONE IS RESPONSIBLE FOR COST

One of the biggest problems contributing to the high cost of medical services is that none of the participants will take or share responsibility for the costs.

The "NOT ME CIRCLE" shows how all the healthcare participants avoid the responsibility for costs.

"Not Me Circle" Excuses

Insurance companies claim, "It's not my fault"

Insurance companies claim they simply provide the employee benefits the employer wants. If the insurance company attempts to curtail cost by reducing claim payments or restricting benefits, the employees and employers complain. In the past, costs have not been a factor, only the improvement of benefits.

The employer claims, "It's not my fault"

Employers blame the insurance company, hospitals and doctors for charging too much, but employees want more benefits, and more coverage. Employers are reluctant to honestly discuss healthcare cost with employees. Some employers use an annual benefits statement to show the employee the company cost of healthcare benefits. The impact of these statements is small, however, because it is difficult for an employee to think of the $4,000 to $10,000 company medical insurance cost as their money. Until an employee can see the medical cost expense as his own money, no action will occur.

To illustrate the concept, consider a consumer's reaction to increases for automobile insurance. The buyer of automobile insurance is requesting a mandated 20 percent rate reduction in certain states. The national average automobile policy is only $500 per year. The consumer is fighting to get a $100 reduction per year. Compare this to the 1988 national average employer medical benefits cost per employee of $2,100, $2,600 in 1989 and $3,100 in 1990. Employer medical benefits cost *increased* $500 per employee in *one year*. The one year *increase* in employer medical cost was equal to the *total* cost of automobile insurance. What did the employee do? Did he request a rate reduction? No. Most employees were not even aware of this large increase and don't care because it *isn't their money.*

Why would buyers fight for a $100 decrease on a $500 car insurance expense and yet willingly accept a $500 *increase* on a $2,600 employer medical expense? It is because employer medical insurance cost is not viewed as employee money. The increase or the total program cost is meaning less to the employee.

Many employers have developed and installed wellness programs to help educate the employee to adopt a healthier lifestyle. These programs address lifestyle changes, exercise programs, fatty foods, cholesterol and stress management. They appear to be successful because the United States population seems to be getting healthier and more health conscious. Yet, medical costs continue to escalate at 10 percent to 30 percent per year, even while hospital admissions decline, *i.e.,* fewer people are getting sick.

Doesn't it make sense for employers to take the next step, and implement educational programs for employees who become sick and must visit a medical provider? Maybe an educational program of this type would encourage employees to take a more active role when they enter the medical system. Employers haven't asked the employee to change their medical buying habits. Instead, the employer has developed employee communication material indicating all the benefits that are provided at "no charge." Isn't it time the employer asked the employee to take responsibility for controlling costs? The employee is on the front line and they are incurring the charges.

Hospitals claim, "It's not me"

Hospitals blame the employer, the patient and the doctor who demand the best quality medical service money can buy. Yet, hospitals won't release quality information to the consumer, such as mortality rates, infection rates, number of times the hospital has done a procedure, so the consumer can make a quality judgement.

Hospitals have had to provide the best facilities and testing equipment to recruit doctors to their hospital. They have not had to deliver the best quality of care to the patient, but rather provide the best equipment and facilities, so the doctor can practice his trade. If the hospital does not have the most modern facilities and on-site office space, doctors may admit their patients to a competitor and the hospital will lose important revenue.

It would appear that hospitals want to be judged by the quality of their tools rather than patient outcomes.

Employees blame everyone

Employees blame insurance companies, employers, doctors and hospitals. Yet employees do not shop for medical services, or ask about quality, they simply present themselves to the healthcare system with the attitude:

> "I don't know what's wrong with me;
> I don't know your qualifications
> but I trust you,
> do whatever is necessary and
> charge whatever you want."

Employees feel access to medical services are a *right* for which they share *no* cost *responsibilities.* When an employee consumes medical services with insurance, he quickly forgets that it is his insurance premium dollars which pay the bill. Rather, he feels it is his right to get as much as he can because it's the insurance company's money. The same applies if the employee believes the care is free (no charge to patient), because at that point there is no incentive to control cost.

It would seem that the American public consumes medical services with the same attitude that teenagers exhibit when they spend their parents' money to buy designer jeans or business people traveling on a corporate expense account. Cost is not a concern, until they start to spend their own hard earned money. Then they become much more value conscious.

The American public buys medical services with no concern for cost or value. Until the public has to spend its own money for medical services, it will not be value conscious.

The lack of concern about costs by the participants of the "not me circle" has lead to tremendous cost increases.

Professional Answers

The professionals (insurance companies, benefit consultants, doctors/hospitals and HMOs) have all tried to control cost through:

Health Maintenance Organizations (HMO)

Preferred Provider Organizations (PPO)

benefit plan designs to encourage the use of low cost nonhospital facilities

encourage use of low cost outpatient facilities

require second opinions

require precertification before hospitalization

increased cost sharing by the employee

and most recently, the new managed care programs which attempt to regulate the provider.

However, based on our past experience of professional intervention (costs have increased 10 percent to 30 percent each year for the last ten years), it appears the professionals cannot effectively control cost without active help from the employee.

With the advent of the new "managed care" concept, the health services industry will become very similar to the military/industrial complex, only we will have a medical provider/insurance company complex. With the "managed care" concept the medical providers and insurance companies join forces to control cost. The combination of the two benefiting forces hasn't reduced cost in the military/industrial complex, but rather has produced some notable excesses. The military/industrial experience should cause some concern for the healthcare consumer with the new medical provider/ insurance company complex. (Is there really any difference between a $650 toilet seat in an airplane and $3.50 for aspirin in the hospital?)

One of the problems which can occur with a "managed care" program is that the provider network used by the insurance company becomes an integral part of the marketing program. As such the insurance companies must always consider medical provider reactions to any benefit changes or reductions that are made. If the insurance company attempts to force difficult cost control changes upon the medical providers, it is possible that the medical providers may rebel and leave. The insurance company then will lose a very effective marketing tool — the network of discounted medical providers.

There is also an inherent problem in expecting organizations who profit from the medical services (hospitals, doctors, and insurance companies) to reduce or control cost.

As an illustration, compare the front page headlines of *Business Insurance* that appeared one week apart:

"Health Plan Rates Rise 20%"	**8/20/90**
"Health Insurer Earnings Peak"	**8/27/90**

The first told employers to expect an average 20 percent medical premium increase next year. The second states that the profits of the largest "managed care" insurance company were up 90.2 percent.

Despite this, the "managed care" concept is still the best program in the healthcare industry, since it provides the lowest consumer cost from discounts provided by the hospitals, doctors and labs. If your insurance company does not provide a "managed care" program the insurance company has to pay "retail" prices while the "managed care" program pays "wholesale." It is unfortunate that a nationwide "managed care" program is not available that covers every city and state. In many rural areas the consumer is virtually "held hostage" by the medical community. There is not enough healthcare competition and the providers do not have to reduce their rates; it will not increase their volume. Therefore very few rural healthcare providers join managed care programs.

Healthcare provider reaction to an insurance company's attempt to control cost can be illustrated with a rubber surgical glove full of air (money). Think of the inflated surgical glove with all five fingers inflated. The insurance company pushes one of the fingers with a "new improved cost containment program." The air (money) simply transfers from one area to another as providers react to the insurance design changes. Even the federal government experiences problems with this bag of air (money). January 1, 1991 a law took effect which stated that all state Medicaid programs must receive the "best price" drug manufacturers offered other large purchasers. The Veterans Administration Hospitals most generally received the "best price" which then also had to be provided to state Medicaid programs. In 1991 the Veterans Administration unit cost of insulin increased 40 percent from one manufacturer. Pain killers increased 900 percent from $5.11 to $47.60 and an ulcer medication increased 200 percent from $16.92 to $34.29.

The intent of the law was to reduce the drug cost for one federal program, Medicare; which it did. But the cost to the Veterans Administration Hospitals increased (punch the glove in one spot and the air moves to another).

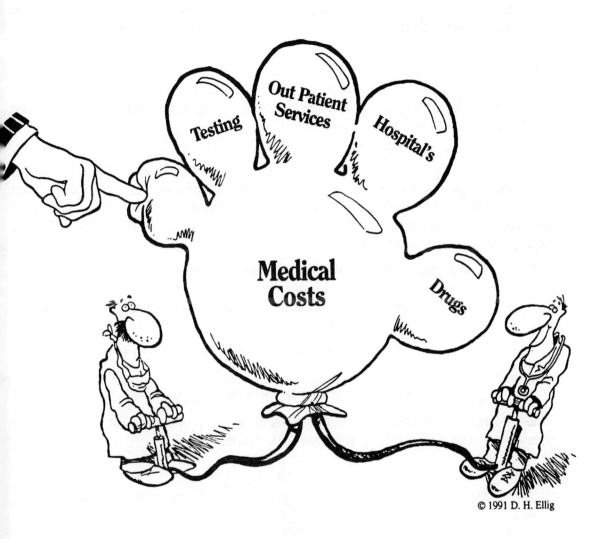

© 1991 D. H. Ellig

Mandated Benefits & More Providers

SUPPLY/DEMAND PLAYERS CONFUSING

If the "not me circle" illustrates that no one is responsible for cost, it also suggests another question, *"Who is the payor of medical services?"*

The "not me circle" also makes it very difficult to determine who the payor is. Is it the employee, employer or the insurance company? Who demands healthcare services? Who supplies healthcare services? This confusion leads to one of the unique features in the medical services industry — the lack of identification of the supply side and demand side players.

In most industries, supply and demand is easily defined, but not so in the healthcare services industry. In the healthcare services industry, at first blush we think the supply side of medical services is the hospitals and doctors and the demand side is the patient. But within the "not me circle" there are other participants and, at any given time, participants may switch sides and be either on the supply side or the demand side.

To illustrate how confusing it is for all the participants consider the following:

— The *employer supplies* the health insurance to the employees who *demand* coverage.

— The *employer demands* the *insurance company supply* the best healthcare coverage.

— The *patient demands* medical services be *supplied* by the *doctor.*

— The *doctors demand* the *hospitals supply* the best care for their patients and the best tools to practice their trade.

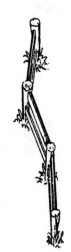

SUPPLY	DEMAND
Employer	Employee
Insurance Company	Employer
Doctor	Patient (Employee)
Hospital	Doctor

In a normal supply/demand model the group demanding services is also the payor. Three out of four of the groups in the above model on the demand side don't *pay the bills.* You can see the problem in the healthcare delivery system, only one group pays the bills, the employer.

If a simple change was made — to have the employee pay more for medical services when they are delivered — it would change the demand side considerably. The result would then be three out of four of the demand groups paying the bills, a more traditional model.

It may seem that employee wouldn't want to pay more for medical services, but if given the choice between paying more for their insurance premium or more for the visit to the healthcare provider, most will choose to pay more when they visit. The reason is very simple — healthcare premiums must be paid every month, even if not used. Healthcare providers are only paid when a visit is required. If employers will review their claims experience, they will find that most (90 percent) of their employees do not have catastrophic medical claims (over $5,000). What this indicates is that most of the employees do not benefit from the medical plan for which the employer is paying large sums of money.

If in the future employers attempt to transfer premium cost to the employees they will find more and more employees dropping the insurance because most of the employees do not use the benefit and do not want to pay for it. A recent survey showed that 60 percent of the employees would pay a maximum of $1,000 a year for their medical benefits. This survey indicates that the value placed on health insurance by employees is considerably different than the value placed on health insurance by the employer ($3,100).

MARKETING RULES ARE DIFFERENT

With the confusion of supply and demand among the individuals in the medical services industry, it is easy to understand why no one will take responsibility for cost. From this confusion the medical services industry has developed unique market features. We are listing only a few of the marketing features enjoyed by the medical services industry:

Prices Not Published

The healthcare services industry is probably the only industry in the United States which does not provide a consumer price list and where the consumer does not ask about price. If the healthcare consumer does dare to inquire about prices, they are given suspicious looks, thought of as odd and probably won't be given prices because even the provider doesn't know the total cost.

Consumer Not Viewed as Payor

No one is held accountable for cost at the point of purchase. Cost is not considered until the insurance company requests a large rate adjustment 12 months after the costs have been incurred. Even then, cost is considered only in aggregate, not in detail for each individual purchase. This is accountability after the fact.

Since the consumer does not pay for services, the industry enjoys the benefit of never having to discuss prices versus service provided. The healthcare provider very rarely has to justify the price for its service and as a result most doctors and hospitals do not know the total treatment plan cost — the cost for *all* the providers of medical services. Doctors do not know the cost of other team members and hospitals can only give rough estimates of treatment plan cost.

Industry Is Not Price Sensitive

Because the consumer is not viewed as the payor, the medical industry can raise prices without fear of consumer reaction. This is not to say the industry is entirely price insensitive. For many years, the media reported yearly increases of hospital room and board rates. The hospitals began to receive unfavorable media attention. What happened? In short order, the hospital room and board rates began to increase very gradually and media attention died. The cost increases were shifted to hospital miscellaneous services which are not available to the public or the media. Now hospital miscellaneous services can be four to seven times the room and board rate, while room and board rates have stabilized.

In the past, the medical provider has been able to increase his prices with little consumer reaction, but today it is becoming more difficult. The federal government, insurance companies, employers and individuals are finally feeling the effect of the high cost of medical services. Costs are being challenged and inefficient facilities are allowed to close.

Hospital Cost Not Challenged by Payor

The major cost of medical services occurs at the hospital. Insurance companies use tables to determine "reasonable" physician and lab service charges. Yet, the most expensive area — hospitals — has no "reasonableness" guidelines. Hospitals may bill any amount for room, board, and miscellaneous charges and it will not be challenged by the insurance companies. They may audit the bill to ensure all listed charges were received by the patient, but "reasonableness" of hospital charges are not challenged. How else can you explain a $1.65 charge for a 3¢ aspirin. Is that reasonable? No other industry could survive the consumer outrage at that kind of a markup.

Some "managed care" programs have negotiated fixed prices via per diem and diagnosis related grouping (DRG) charges. If you are not in a "managed care" program or without insurance, the "reasonable fee" is whatever the hospital wants to charge.

80 Percent Off Sale

This is one of the few industries in which the consumer can automatically take 80 percent off the price of services. Everyday is sale day. Most benefit plans pay 80 percent or 100 percent of the cost of services. The consumer only pays 20 percent. Think of how many other industries could benefit by presenting an 80 percent discount to their consumers. Do you suppose the demand in other industries would increase?

Quality Not Possible to Determine

Doctors and hospitals refuse to supply information to the consumer that would allow the patient to determine the quality of provided services. Doctors refuse to provide references to patients who have undergone treatment to help new patients determine the quality of services provided. Questioning one doctor about another doctor's qualifications results in nebulous statements that make it impossible for the consumer to make an informed decision.

Hospitals do not release information about mortality, infection, complication rates or the number of times a procedure has been performed, making it impossible for the consumer to judge quality at their facility.

All Medical Providers Are Created Equal

Without quality information the consumer can only presume all providers are equal. This is *not true*. Without quality data it is impossible for the consumer to make a value judgement of provider services. As a result, consumers can be treated by a substandard provider without their knowledge and typically discover it only after unsatisfactory care or outcomes, which is *too late*.

Unfortunately, due to the lack of quality and price information, the consumer presumes all providers to be equal, which is a mistake.

Independent Doctors versus Employees

Most industries have manufacturing sites with buildings, testing equipment and facilities that are staffed with employees. This is done to control performance and cost. Yet, in the medical industry, hospitals supply only the facilities, equipment and support staff for use by very independent doctors who practice their profession using the hospital equipment and staff. The anesthesiologist, radiologist, pathologist and surgeon simply enter the hospital and use the equipment while practicing their trade and then leave.

What other industry operates this way?

Why doesn't the hospital simply employ surgeons, radiologists, and anesthesiologists so that the hospital can better control quality and cost?

Trainees Are Paid as Much as Old Pros

This is probably the only industry in the world which allows a trainee to charge as much for his inexperience as an experienced person. New surgeons and doctors charge and are paid as much as the surgeon who has practiced 20 years. The only other professions that allow trainees to earn as much as experienced people are those professions which operate purely on commission.

New Business Rate Failures Are Not Feared

It is estimated that 5 out of 10 new businesses started in the United States will fail within the first 3 years. When was the last time you saw a new physician suffer a financial business failure? It appears the system is designed to guarantee a new physician financial success.

Excess Capacity

The average hospital occupancy rate in the United States is 58 percent. Some hospitals continue to keep their doors open while at 25 percent capacity. Very few industries can operate profitably at 58 percent capacity or be allowed to simply raise prices to cover the expense of the 42 percent surplus capacity and also continue to add new facilities.

In most economic systems, surplus capacity causes a decrease in price. This is not true in the medical service industries. Consider what happens when a second hospital enters a small community. Instead of decreasing, prices increase to cover the expenses of the sudden surplus bed capacity, duplication of services and equipment. Both hospitals must provide the latest equipment to attract the limited number of doctors who admit patients that generate hospital revenue.

The number of doctors in the United States has nearly doubled since 1960. Some sources indicate this suggests an oversupply of doctors. With an oversupply of doctors we would expect the price to go down. But the cost per surgery increases because each doctor performs fewer surgeries. Compare that to what happens when three competitive stores locate at one street intersection — a price war results. In most industries, if you have more competitors, the price goes down. This is not true in the medical services industry.

Think about it. Have you ever heard of a gallbladder surgery price war or a heart bypass surgery price war when a new physician enters the community?

Rather than a price decrease, prices go up to compensate for the reduced number of surgeries each additional physician will be able to perform. Could this also lead to the occasional unnecessary surgery being performed?

Duplication versus Specialization

Even though there are many hospital services and equipment duplications, there is very little community effort to encourage hospitals to offer specialized treatment programs (*i.e.*, one hospital for heart, one for cancer, one for neurology, etc., and several general low cost hospitals), or to limit the amount of expensive testing equipment).

Well People Pay Nearly as Much as Sick People

The average cost of medical insurance for an average family of a mother, father and child is $4,000 to $7,000 per year. The most common benefit plan protects the individual with a maximum medical expense of $1,300. (A $300 deductible and 20 percent to $5,000.) It seems strange that it costs $4,000 to $7,000 if you remain well, and only an additional $1,300 if medical expenses cost $30,000, $200,000 or $1,000,000. Wouldn't it make more sense if it only cost $1,300 to remain well and $4,000 to $7,000 if you were sick? The sick can always arrange to pay their bills with monthly payments, rather than have all pay high insurance premiums.

LACK OF QUALITY DEFINITION

It is a common belief that the United States has the highest quality of medical services in the world. We probably do, but the problem is that only the medical insiders, doctors, nurses, and hospital administrators know who the best quality providers are. You and I, as the medical consumer, don't have the slightest idea who is the best healthcare provider, or more importantly, who should be avoided.

Healthcare providers normally measure quality of medical services by patient satisfaction, indicated by the manner in which services are delivered and the availability of high tech diagnostic equipment. However, if quality of medical services are measured by other factors, perhaps the United States does not provide the best quality of medical services. Consider the following as indicators of medical quality:

— Life Expectancy: Despite the fact that the United States has the highest cost for healthcare in the world it does not have the highest life expectancy. Other countries with lower medical costs have higher life expectancies.

— Infant Mortality: The United States has a higher infant mortality rate than other countries with lower healthcare cost.

— Population Covered by Medical Insurance: The United States has the largest number of people not covered by health insurance among the industrialized nations. We currently have approximately 33 to 37 million people not covered by health insurance.

— Access to Health Treatment: The United States has wonderful access to healthcare providers if you have insurance. If you do not have health insurance, access is very difficult to achieve.

— High Tech Diagnostic Equipment: The United States, without a doubt, has the greatest number of high tech diagnostic equipment such as MRIs and CT scanners.

— Cost: The United States has the highest cost for healthcare in the world.

If we review all of these issues, it becomes obvious that when the American public is told that the United States has the highest quality of medical care "they" must be referring to our access to high tech diagnostic equipment and cost, rather than the other important issues of infant mortality, life expectancy, population coverage and access to providers.

It is interesting to note that in the United States our definition of high quality medical care is defined by the tools we use, rather than the outcome of the product. What other industry measures the quality of their product by the tools they use, rather than the product they produce?

CONCLUSION

The United States is rapidly approaching a healthcare crisis. As costs escalate, more and more people and employers will reject the high insurance premium costs and chose to be without insurance protection, resulting in higher rates for those who remain insured.

How important is high tech medical care if we cannot pay for it or have access to it? We have the technology to replace kidneys in newborns, but most of us couldn't afford the treatment without medical insurance. Medical technology is increasing faster than our ability to pay for it. People without medical insurance who are unable to pay before services are unable to have a simple cyst removed or undergo serious surgery. They are regularly, flatly denied medical treatment by healthcare providers. Is it right that we can spend millions to save one life and deny basic medical access to millions?

Who is the ultimate payor?

We all know it's you and me.   We are currently losing wages, paying increasing Social Security and income taxes to pay for medical services. Until the medical services cost dilemma is resolved, we must be more proactive with our medical providers to help reduce cost and improve quality or we may lose our ability to freely choose our medical services.

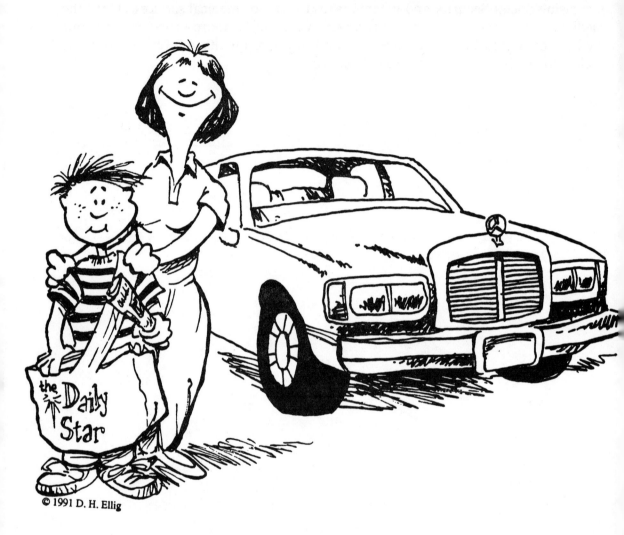

© 1991 D. H. Ellig

"My Son, The Paper Boy"

CHAPTER 18

WHAT IF . . .
NEWSPAPERS AND MEDICAL SERVICES WERE DELIVERED THE SAME WAY

The medical services industry operates in a unique economic environment. This may best be illustrated by applying medical economic characteristics to another industry and observing the effect the characteristics would have on that industry.

The newspaper publishing industry is used here since it easily lends itself to a simple comparison that everyone can understand. Nearly everyone in the United States has used newspaper publishing services either for subscription or advertising. This two-industry comparison uses some poetic or writer's license. As such, it is not entirely accurate. It is presented solely to illustrate the unique economic environment that the medical services industry enjoys.

Cast of Characters

Hospitals	Played by	Newspaper Publishers
Doctors	Played by	Reporters/Paper Carriers
Diagnostic Equipment	Played by	Reporters' Equipment (Desk Top Publishing)
Medical Insurance Rates	Played by	Newspaper Subscription Rates
Medical Cost	Played by	Advertising Rates
Insurance Company	Played by	Third Party

First there would no longer be only one or two newspaper publishers in major metropolitan areas. Almost all major cities would have 5, 15 or 20 newspaper publishers.

The increased competition would not result in a cost decrease, but rather a cost increase. The duplication of equipment and facilities would ultimately result in excess capacity and there would also be a few nonprofit publishers with the same lavish equipment and facilities as the for-profit companies.

The publishers would be able to decrease their subscription rates by 80 percent to the subscriber and limit an advertiser's cost to a maximum of $1,300 a year. (The advertiser would still have to pay a deductible of the first $300 advertising cost and 20 percent of the next $5,000.) A third party would pay the other 80 percent — someone with lots of money. The third party's financial condition would be as solid as a rock.

This decrease in cost to the advertiser would probably result in increased advertising usage. The advertiser, who had advertised monthly with a small one-column, black-and-white ad, would now be enticed to advertise weekly or daily with a four-page, four-color glossy insert. Since someone else was now paying most of the advertising expense, cost would not be a consideration.

The reduced advertising cost would be especially beneficial to newborn businesses and old failing businesses as "heroic" advertising efforts would be provided to save the business.

The reporters and newspaper carriers would not be employees of the publisher, but would be free to practice their profession at any newspaper facility. The newspaper publisher would provide the facility and staff to assist the reporters in practicing their profession.

Because of this new relationship between newspaper publishers and reporters, and the need for the publisher to fill its newspapers with stories, the publisher would invest in the most modern equipment and technologies to encourage reporters to file their stories with the publisher's newspaper.

Occasionally, although newspaper publishers would do their utmost to provide the most modern facilities and equipment, groups of reporters would also buy technically advanced and expensive equipment. The reporters would then use their own equipment to layout articles and add the equipment cost to their fees to increase their cash flow, even though their personal equipment duplicated equipment already provided by the publishers.

The incomes of the reporters and newspaper carriers would increase astronomically because the publishers would no longer have the responsibility of paying for reporting services. The third party would pay and pass the cost along in rate increases. No one would question prices for stories and reporters wouldn't even discuss prices with the publisher. The third party would pay 80 percent for reporting services and home delivery of newspapers.

Think of the result:

* Newspapers would become an ideal employee benefit and unions would bargain for home delivery.

* Colleges would recruit only the best and brightest to be reporters and paper carriers and admissions would be limited.

* Mothers would introduce their sons as "my son the paper boy."

* On rainy days, the papers would be delivered under domed silver platters tied with a velvet bow by a paper carrier driving a Mercedes Benz.

* If a home owner had a complaint about the delivery service or wet newspapers, he would have to complain to the State Board of Paper Carriers. This state board would be made up of 12 paper carriers who would review the complaint because the process of delivering papers would be too complicated for the lay person to understand. Other paper boys would not testify against the paper boy under review because of the fear of slander, libel, court cost and the thought, "there but by the grace of God go I."

With the newspaper publishers operating in this new economic environment, the United States would have the best quality newspaper services in the world, but would cost two or three times more than the cost of newspaper publishing in Great Britain or Canada. When the largest advertiser, the United States government, recognized the high cost, it would reduce its advertising. As a result, cost would be shifted to the private sector and would increase dramatically. The cost of advertising and home delivery would escalate so sharply that business and homeowners would complain. Soon a large portion of the population would not be able to afford the newspaper.

When people would ask reporters and publishers why the United States doesn't have a newspaper delivery system similar to that of Canada or Great Britain, the response would be that the quality of newspapers and advertising would be reduced. Papers would be printed on newsprint rather than glossy paper. Ads would be black and white rather than four color, and one-eighth page in size, versus full page. Also, the ink would rub off on your hands and your paper would have to be delivered by bicycle and wrapped in plastic.

But wouldn't we still get the same news, just delivered in a different fashion in a different system?

Health Care Crisis Solutions

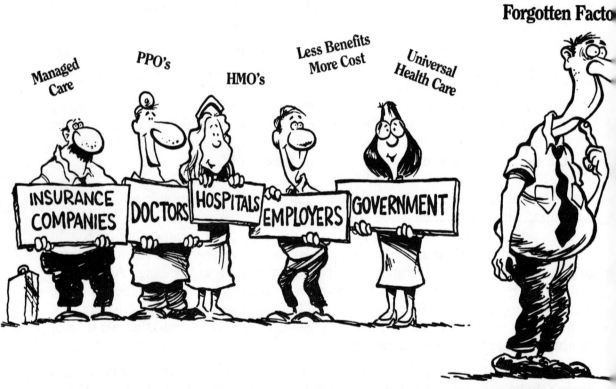

Patient, Consumer,
Employee

CHAPTER 19

THE GRAND DESIGN

As we all know, the United States is facing a severe crisis in its healthcare delivery system. Without some changes, medical care in the United States will become unaffordable in the very near future (it is already unaffordable for 32 to 37 million people). Quite obviously the healthcare system must change.

The entire content of this book is based on the premise that the consumer (patient) has not been actively involved in the issues of quality, service and price. This information has been withheld from the consumer, either by design, lack of knowledge or motivation. If the consumer does not become involved in issues of quality, price and services, someone else will, and currently that looks like the government. If the government becomes involved, all the participants in the healthcare delivery system will loose something. If the American public wishes to maintain its right to free choice of healthcare providers, we all must take more responsibility.

We are, therefore, taking the liberty of outlining a "grand design" for a change in the United States healthcare delivery system based on consumer involvement and information access. It is understood that this may be presumptuous and that some of the ideas may be unworkable and wishful thinking. Nevertheless, for the last 50 years, consumer (patient) involvement has never been addressed as a possible solution for the healthcare delivery system crisis. We believe that some of these precepts and concepts should be tried before we have a national healthcare delivery system. The systems suggested currently exist, are available and operating. They need only be distributed and implemented. The concept of healthcare consumer education works. A Swiss study which provided prospective patients with information concerning hysterectomies resulted in 25 percent fewer hysterectomies.

EMPLOYER'S ROLE

Employers need to carefully consider this statement:

**You have reduced their benefits,
increased their cost,
what's next?**

If employers are to pass additional cost to the employee, either by higher premiums or fewer benefits, they need to provide employees the tools to manage their increased costs.

Employers need to take an active lead position as healthcare consumer advocates, since they have the greatest interest. **Their money is funding the healthcare delivery system.** The cost to adopt a healthcare consumer education program as shown would be less than 1 percent of their medical premiums, a small price compared with annual increases of 25 percent.

Medical Library — Employers should provide employees access to a well-stocked consumer medical library, including books, periodicals and consumer newsletters.

Employers also may want to consider sharing the subscription cost of disease specific magazines for those employees with long-term illnesses such as diabetes and heart conditions. These magazines provide the latest information concerning treatments, product evaluation and lifestyle tips. The subscription cost is only $12 to $24 a year, much less expensive than one visit to the doctor.

Database Access — The medical library should provide employees access to medical databases, such as Medline and the FDA recall database.

In addition, they should purchase drug software programs that allow the employee to research the interactions and reactions of drugs, plus printout cautions and warnings in plain English.

Cost Sharing — Employers should offer a reduced benefit plan design. A reduced benefits plan is actually *more equitable,* as the employee who uses the benefit would pay more when they incur medical expenses, rather than *all* employees paying more in medical premiums. A 50/50 cost sharing will cause the employee to become a *buyer* of medical services than simply a *consumer* of medical services. The total maximum employee out-of-pocket expense should be such that the employee is still protected against catastrophic medical claims (only 5 to 10 percent of the employees have medical expenses over $5,000). Many employees would rather have money in their pocket today, than pay high health insurance premiums. Most would rather pay medical costs when they are incurred rather than in advance with high medical premiums. They can always negotiate monthly provider payments thereby *paying after* an event rather than *paying before* an event which may or may not happen.

Which is it?

Pay in Advance

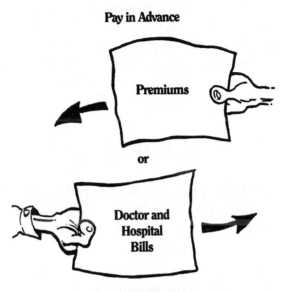

Pay when Incurred?

Education Programs — Employers should implement educational programs with videos and newsletters that help the employees become better healthcare consumers.

**Employees incur claims . . .
insurance companies pay claims . . .
who can really control cost?**

Incentives — Employer health plans should be designed to reward employees who shop for medical services, both on quality and price issues. Those employees who have a healthier lifestyle should receive a premium discount.

Encourage Use of Doctors and Hospitals — Employers should encourage employees to use healthcare providers who encourage consumer participation by providing prices, quality and truly provide informed consent information before treatment.

Donations to Libraries — Employers should donate money to their local libraries to fund medical database access. For less than $10,000 per year they could provide their community free access to medical information. What a gift!

Donations to Hospitals — Large employers contribute funds to hospitals at hospital charity balls. Employers may want to consider donating funds and supporting those hospitals that are receptive to their employees' needs, such as true informed consent, providing true quality information and drug testing of doctors and staff. In this way employers can make a statement that they care about quality of care and are willing to support those hospitals that provide it.

A note of caution, employers must continue to offer insurance plans. If employees are given a choice between medical insurance or cash, a majority will choose cash and not buy medical insurance resulting in more people without insurance and low participation (mostly the sick) in employer plans. Also, a recent survey showed that 70 percent of employees would pay less than $1,000 for medical insurance, if the cost exceeded $1,000 they would drop the insurance. The employee's value judgment of medical insurance is greatly distorted from the actual 1990 average employer cost of $3,100.

DOCTOR'S ROLE

Doctor's offices of the future should become information sources for the patient. Currently the patient spends 15 to 45 minutes waiting for physician services. Why not use that time to provide consumer health information?

If a physician voluntarily adhered to the first six points listed below, the practice would grow, because patients will seek doctors who provide consumer information services and whose qualifications are prominently displayed. (If you build it, they will come!)

Medical Library — The physician should provide access to a consumer medical library stocked with consumer medical books on medical testing, self-diagnosis, drugs, a medical dictionary and consumer medical newsletters.

Computer Terminals — Doctor's offices should have computer terminals available for patient access to drug and medical databases and to print out selected information.

It also would be appropriate for the physician to have a service price list that the patient could access.

Qualify Notification — What do you suppose would happen if your physician posted his qualifications as outlined in the "Ask Your Doctor" chapter, and helped the patient qualify the other providers such as doctor referrals, labs and hospitals. That would be providing a service!

Drug Test — Doctors should voluntarily submit to drug testing for themselves and their staff and perhaps have a poster stating the office is "certified drug free."

Informed Consent — Physicians should voluntarily adhere to the informed consent doctrine by supplying patients with full, written documentation of the risks, complications, benefits and alternative treatments. Patients should be informed that complications may occur, are expected and can occur without negligence by the doctor.

Recall Warnings Posted — Why not have a recall board where FDA actions, warnings and recalls of drugs and medical devices could be posted so that patients would be informed of health hazards. This seems like an easy way to disseminate important patient information to patients, who in turn will inform friends and relatives.

Treatment Methods — Physicians should first treat patients as human beings rather than as a disease to be cured.

Use Physician Assistants and Nurse Practitioners — The more common illnesses and accidents should be treated by physician's assistants and nurse practitioners. Doctors should be free to treat those patients with more complex conditions. This will allow the physician to fully utilize his training and experience where it is most beneficial.

Patient Access to Physician Databank — Doctors should support opening the physician databank to the healthcare consumer. This would relieve them of the guilt of knowing that some physicians shouldn't be "practicing" medicine.

As innovative as these ideas may sound, they are all supported by AMA Ethics Standards.

HOSPITAL ROLE

Hospitals should voluntarily provide information to the patients to make an informed decision about the quality of service at the hospital. Of course only the best hospitals would provide this information but their patient census would increase.

Quality Issues — The hospitals should voluntarily provide information to the patient on the following issues:

JACHO Accreditation

Radiology Accreditation

Mortality, Infection and Complication Rates

Number of Board Certified Doctors to Total Doctors

Number of RNs to Total Nursing Staff

Occupancy Rates

Drug Testing — Hospitals should require drug testing of the surgery staff, including doctors. The hospital surgical team makes more life and death decisions on a daily basis than any business in the United States. Take a stand, do something for the patient for whom you provide a service.

Cost Estimates — Hospitals should provide cost estimates for the hospital stay. Software to provide cost estimates is now available, hospitals currently have 3 to 6 billing systems in place already to provide different prices to different payors, *i.e.,* Medicare, Medicaid, PPO, HMO and retail.

Consumer Information — Hospitals should have a consumer information center. This center would include a consumer medical library and computer retrieval of medical studies. Many patients and family members do not understand what the doctors and hospital staff are saying, doing or why. If a medical information center were available, it would be used, it could even be a revenue source for the hospital. Why not allow patients to use, for a fee, the computer retrieval services and staff currently available to doctors, or sell consumer medical books in the hospital gift shop?

Patient Access to Records — Hospitals should allow patients access to their own medical records, withholding information creates fear, tension, and reduces the patient's ability to contribute to their own treatment.

Lay People on Boards — Hospitals should ask for volunteer lay person representation on the peer review and credentialing process boards.

It has been said, *"War is too important to leave to the Generals."* The United States has reached the point where *"Healthcare is too important to leave to the doctors and hospitals."* Healthcare policies have been developed to protect the interest of the healthcare provider - very little has been formulated to protect the patient. It is time for the consumer to get involved! Maybe they can make some of the decisions that doctors and hospitals find difficult.

GOVERNMENT

It should be acknowledged that the government has been very successful in controlling the cost of the healthcare delivery for its Medicare and Medicaid programs by dictating the prices it will pay. The problem is that it has been too good and caused prices to spiral in the private sector. It may now be appropriate for the government to do something for the private sector. It is time to make consumer information available so that the consumer can make an informed buying decision based on value judgments. It would seem that it would be less costly to provide information to the patient than to fund large programs to control providers and prices. The government also may benefit by dissemination of consumer information, since it currently pays almost one-half of the United States healthcare cost.

The government should consider that

It is better to teach how to consume than to regulate consumption.

The following are suggested areas of government involvement:

Medicare — Healthcare Provider Reimbursement — The government should continue developing the Medicare reimbursement schedules for physicians and hospitals that recognize the value of cognitive physician services and rewards hospitals that are financially well-managed.

Medicare should reimburse for the services of physician's assistants and nurse practitioners. It may be that doctors don't employ physician's assistants or nurse practitioners because Medicare does not cover their services and Medicare reimbursement can be 40 percent to 60 percent of a physician's revenue. Currently Medicare pays for physician's assistants and nurse practitioners services only in rural areas. Why not all areas?

Malpractice Reforms — Don't do it until the doctors and hospitals have demonstrated a good faith attempt to control malpractice claims by implementing a "true" informed consent form upon which is recorded all the information suggested by the informed consent doctrine. A properly documented *written record* of explicit risks and expected outcomes would greatly improve understanding and lead to fewer malpractice claims.

An excellent compromise on the medical malpractice tort reform issue would be to grant tort relief *only* to those doctors and hospitals that provide the patient *written documentation* of the risk probabilities and complications, plus all the information that doctors *say* they provided when they signed the Informed Consent form.

This compromise would provide two benefits; the doctors and hospitals would get their tort relief and the patient would get the full written information necessary to make an informed decision.

Many claims result from patient lack of understanding of the treatment plan and outcomes. Is it possible that if the patient were truly informed and patient information was properly recorded in writing that malpractice claims would decline sharply?

A majority (over 50 percent) of physician malpractice claims result from misdiagnosis or failure to diagnose. Very few claims result from true technical negligence.

Fifty percent of hospital claims are from doctors who sue the hospital for restraint of trade when hospital admitting privileges are denied. Why change torts to protect the healthcare delivery system from itself? Why not provide legislation that would outline when a hospital may deny admitting privileges.

Physician's Databank — Insist that the healthcare consumer be allowed access to the physician databank, which contains physicians who have been disciplined. AMA ethics state that doctors should "Strive to expose those physicians deficient in character and competence . . ." and "to seek changes in those requirements that are contrary to the best interest of the patient." AMA ethics would seem to support release of the information to the patient.

Patient Self-Determination Act — This act currently requires Medicare and Medicaid healthcare providers to provide the patient with written notification of their right to refuse service. It should be expanded to assure that healthcare providers provide written notification of the informed consent doctrine, wherein the patient is informed provided explicitly written information about the treatment risk, consequences, complications and alternative treatments.

Medline — Government should continue to fund the Medline database, since it is the least expensive and most complete source of medical information.

Medical Records — States that have laws which restrict patients access to their own medical records should be encouraged to remove that restriction. It certainly isn't protecting the patient, especially when the patient must provide an oral history for each new doctor. Doctors know oral patient history is their most unreliable source. It may be a contributing factor to the doctor's reliance on extensive testing.

Drugs — Drug Warnings — Drug manufacturers should be required to provide patient information in print size that is legible and written in a language that is simply understood. Some states require insurance companies to provide easy to read insurance contracts, why not drug warnings?

WARNING

This paragraph is a reprint of the above text. The printing above is an example of the actual print size of a drug manufacturer's warning. The drug warning concerned drug interactions, carcinogens, a warning for consumption during pregnancy and for nursing mothers, pediatric use instructions, adverse reactions and probable causal relationships greater than one percent, incidents less than one percent, effect of overdosage, dosage and administration, how supplied and drug company name. How can you warn a consumer if the print is so small it can't be read without a magnifying glass?

This paragraph is a reprint of the above text. The printing above is an example of the actual print size of a drug manufacturer's warning. The drug warning concerned drug interactions, carcinogens, a warning for consumption during pregnancy and for nursing mothers, pediatric use instructions, adverse reactions and probable causal relationships greater than one percent, incidents less than one percent, effect of overdosage, dosage and administration, how supplied and drug company name. How can you warn a consumer if the print is so small it can't be read without a magnifying glass?

Therapeutic Gain — The FDA should require drug labeling of the *therapeutic gain* of new drugs so doctors and consumers can make a value judgment of "me too" drugs brought to market. Why should the consumer pay up to 10 times more for a new drug that offers no therapeutic improvement or gain? It also would be appropriate to change the rating code from A, B and C so that doctors and consumers do not *confuse therapeutic gain* with *therapeutic equivalency.*

Post Prices — Pharmacies in canada are required to post the prices of the top 20 most frequently prescribed drugs on a 2' by 3' sign. This allows the consumer to shop for the best price. The cost for a tranquilizer prescription is $48.00 in the United States and $7.00 in Canada. It must work, the consumer does shop.

Medical Device Recall — The Government should require medical device manufacturers to notify all patients of any warnings or recalls. It is incomprehensible that the government can require car manufacturers to inform car buyers of automobile recalls and not to require medical device manufacturers to inform patients with their implanted medical devices that their product may be hazardous to the patient's health.

Taxes — Taxes on cigarettes and alcohol should be increased and the funds used to offset Medicare expenses. This concept has been successfully applied in Canada and several other countries with national healthcare systems.

Taxing employer-provided medical benefits is an excellent idea. If employees had to pay taxes on the high cost of employer-provided medical benefits, they would quickly ask the employer to reduce benefits so their taxes would decrease. Less benefits would create more employee cost at time of healthcare provider visits, which would automatically cause more consumer involvement: asking for prices, asking about treatment alternatives and questioning need for testing.

Taxing employer-provided medical benefits would immediately effect consumer involvement in the healthcare industry. Congress, however, will not tax benefits. The combined lobbying of AMA (American Medical Association), AHA (American Hospital Association), insurance companies and labor unions would be too great.

A Better Idea — A "healthcare" IRA — Better than taxing benefits is the implementation of a plan that would allow the employee to self-fund their major medical expenses. Self-funding has worked well for employers (most large employers now self-fund their medical plans). Employers who self-fund their programs take a much more active role in adopting cost control ideas. Maybe the same will happen with employees.

The government should allow employees to set aside a maximum of $1,000, $2,000, $5,000 or $10,000 to pay for major medical expenses. The amounts could be set aside on a tax-free basis, much like IRA or 401(k) contributions, but could only be withdrawn for medical expenses. Any other withdrawal would incur a tax and penalty. Maybe as an incentive, the first $500, $1,000 or $2,000 could be taxed on withdrawal and the remainder withdrawn tax-free. This may increase individual cost awareness.

At first blush Congress may be hesitant to lose a tax base, but loss of this tax base could be much less than continuing to fund increases for healthcare expenses or a national healthcare policy.

Give the consumer the chance to exercise their *"buying"* rights before implementing a national healthcare policy.

It has always been said that the only two sure things in life are death and taxes. In the United States there are only three sure things, large healthcare expenses, death and taxes. You can't leave this place without having major healthcare expenses that can greatly reduce the assets available for the survivor.

EMPLOYEE

Surprising as it may sound, we don't have a *"national"* healthcare crisis, we have a *"personal"* healthcare crisis. If we don't *"personally"* get involved, many of us will be without health insurance.

Employees need to understand that . . .

The right to benefits
has responsibilities.

If the employee does not take the responsibility to be a better healthcare consumer, they will lose their right to benefits.

The employee must remember that they are in a very powerful position when buying medical services. They are dealing with an industry that has too much capacity (hospitals are 58 percent full and there are now twice as many doctors as in 1960). **They need your business.**

The consumer must be provided with information to make an informed decision. Consumer information is supported by case law and the ethical standards of the American Medical Association. The proper information will allow the consumer to make a decision on the necessity of the treatment and a value judgement of services to be provided.

Employees should demand access to medical treatment information. They should know their rights, exercise them and educate themselves.

They should not allow themselves to be talked down to by healthcare providers. Employees are very intelligent, the employer depends on them to make a profit. Employees have put people on the moon, and drive 18-wheel trucks in Los Angeles rush hour traffic. It is simply not appropriate to make statements that the patient cannot understand their medical treatment program or alternatives and it is in direct conflict with informed consent doctrine.

The employee should consider healthcare plans that provide only catastrophic coverage and assume responsibility for the small bills.

SUMMARY

If we are to allow people free access to the medical delivery system, the consumer must be involved. It will require the work of all the participants in the United States healthcare delivery system, the government, the insurance companies, the hospitals, the doctors, the employer and the employees.

Most of the suggestions contained in this chapter fall within the guidelines of the two major healthcare organizations: The American Medical Association and the American Hospital Association. Both of these organizations have position papers outlining steps to address the issue of healthcare.

The American Medical Association's proposal is addressed in "Health Access America." This is a 16-point plan, four of which are:

* Develop proposals that encourage cost-conscious decisions by patients

* Seek innovation in insurance underwriting

* Encourage health promotion by physicians and patients

* Urge expanded federal support for medical education, research and the National Institute of Health to continue progress toward medical breakthroughs

The American Hospital Association also has a position paper called "AHA National Health Strategy Project." Three of the goals addressed in this paper are:

* Insuring high quality healthcare

* Responding to consumer needs

* Sparking innovation

We realize that on the surface these two organizations should probably support the suggestions of the "grand design." It will take great courage on their part, however, to actually support the issues in the "grand design," since an informed consumer might result in less income for their member. These two organizations must make a decision whether they're going to answer to the consumer or to the government.

NOTES

CHAPTER 20

PATH TO GOOD HEALTH

There are a few simple actions that individuals can take to maintain or improve their health. Most are very simple but may require lifestyle changes. Lifestyle changes promote better self-image and help us control some aspects of our lives.

This chapter will address only a few areas but the results can be dramatic and control in these few areas can decrease our risk of heart disease and cancer, the two biggest causes of death in the United States. First a few simple suggestions.

Laugh!!

Take time to relax without interruptions - walk

Exercise 20 minutes per day, three times per week

Do not use any tobacco products

Moderate or no use of alcohol

Don't drink and drive

Always use your seat belt

Remember your mother! Eat your vegetables and fiber. (She was a very modern lady.)

Here are some general guidelines for good health with testing frequencies as suggested by medical organizations.

		<u>Depending on Age</u>
Blood Pressure		Less than 130/85
Cholesterol	Good	Less than 200
	Borderline	200 - 240
	High Risk	Greater than 240
LDL (Bad Cholesterol)	Good	Less than 130
	Borderline	130 - 160
	High Risk	Greater than 160
HDL (Good Cholesterol)	High Risk	Less than 35
Blood Glucose	Good	Less than 120 MGM %
Liver Function GGTP	Good	Less than 35

The American Cancer Society recommends the following testing frequencies. Your cancer risk profile may require certain tests be done more frequently.

<u>Age</u>	<u>20 - 40</u>	<u>40 and Over</u>
Cancer Related Checkup (Thyroid, Oral, Lymph Nodes, etc.)	Every 3 Years	Every Other
Breast		
Doctor	Every 3 Years	Every Year
Self-Exam	Every Month	Every Month
Mammogram	Baseline at 35/40	Every 2 Years 40/49
		Every Year after 50
Uterus		
Pelvic	Every 3 Years	Every Year
Pap Smear	After 2 Negatives	After 2 Negatives
	1 Every 3 Years	1 Every 3 Years
Endometrium Tissue		At Menopause
Colon/Rectum		
Digital Exam		Every Year
Stool Slide		Every Year After 50
Procto Exam		After 2 Negatives
		1 Every 1-3 Years
		After 50
Testicular		
Self Exam	Every Month	Every Month
Skin Cancer	If a Change in Mole or Unusual Skin Condition	
Lung Cancer	X-ray Detection is Not Early Enough — Prevention is Best — Don't Smoke	

Cancer Help Line 1-800-227-2345 (A good source for help/guidance and updated treatment plans.)

Weight tables always generate interest and people are also looking for a weight table which "fits." Therefore, we have provided two weight tables for your convenience.

TABLE 1

Suggested Weight (Without Clothes or Shoes)
(The higher weights generally apply to men, the lower to women.)

Height	19 to 34 Years	35 Years and Over
5'0"	97 — 128	108 — 138
5'1"	101 — 132	111 — 143
5'2"	104 — 137	115 — 148
5'3"	107 — 141	119 — 152
5'4"	111 — 146	122 — 157
5'5"	114 — 150	126 — 162
5'6"	118 — 155	130 — 167
5'7"	121 — 160	134 — 172
5'8"	125 — 164	138 — 178
5'9"	129 — 169	142 — 183
5'10"	132 — 174	146 — 188
5'11"	136 — 179	151 — 194
6'0"	140 — 184	155 — 199
6'1"	144 — 189	159 — 205
6'2"	148 — 195	164 — 210
6'3"	152 — 200	168 — 216
6'4"	156 — 205	173 — 222

United States Food and Drug Administration "Healthy Weights

TABLE 2

Good Fitness Weight*
(Without Shoes in Indoor Clothing)

MEN				WOMEN			
Height	Small Frame	Medium Frame	Large Frame	Height	Small Frame	Medium Frame	Large Frame
5'1"	112 — 120	118 — 129	126 — 141	4'8"	96 — 98	96 — 107	104 — 119
5'2"	115 — 123	121 — 133	129 — 144	4'9"	94 — 101	98 — 110	106 — 122
5'3"	118 — 126	124 — 136	132 — 148	4'10"	96 — 104	101 — 113	109 — 125
5'4"	121 — 129	127 — 139	135 — 152	4'11"	99 — 107	104 — 116	112 — 128
5'5"	124 — 133	130 — 143	138 — 156	5'0"	102 — 110	107 — 119	115 — 131
5'6"	128 — 137	134 — 147	142 — 161	5'1"	105 — 113	110 — 122	118 — 134
5'7"	132 — 141	138 — 152	147 — 166	5'2"	108 — 116	113 — 126	121 — 138
5'8"	136 — 145	142 — 156	151 — 170	5'3"	111 — 119	116 — 130	125 — 142
5'9"	140 — 150	146 — 160	155 — 174	5'4"	114 — 123	120 — 135	129 — 146
5'10"	144 — 154	150 — 165	159 — 179	5'5"	118 — 127	124 — 139	133 — 150
5'11"	148 — 158	154 — 170	164 — 184	5'6"	122 — 131	128 — 143	137 — 154
6'0"	152 — 162	158 — 175	168 — 189	5'7"	126 — 135	132 — 147	141 — 158
6'1"	156 — 167	162 — 180	173 — 194	5'8"	130 — 140	136 — 151	145 — 163
6'2"	160 — 171	167 — 185	178 — 199	5'9"	134 — 144	140 — 155	149 — 168
6'3"	164 — 175	172 — 190	182 — 204	5'10"	138 — 148	144 — 159	153 — 173

*Metropolitan Life

An unscientific method which can be used to determine frame size is to circle your wrist with your thumb and longest finger. If they overlap you have a small frame, if they touch you have a medium frame, if they don't touch you have a large frame. It's a simple unscientific way to answer the question, "What size frame am I?"

CHAPTER 21

CONCLUSION

This book provides the healthcare consumer access to many sources and methods to become more involved in their medical treatment. The human mind, being what it is, retains verbal conversations only for a short time. If all the information you have gathered is retained without written record, it will soon disappear.

It is strongly suggested that you retain a written record of the information you used to make your medical treatment decision. Therefore, listed below are those pieces of information which should be recorded in writing and retained.

GET IT IN WRITING

1) Treatment risk, outcome probabilities and expected benefits
(The Risk Assessment is a good form for recording this data, get as much as you can)

2) Doctor letter releasing medical records and stating that you are to be provided copies of all test results

3) Price estimates (copies of previous bills)

4) Copies of test results

5) Drug warnings, interactions and side effects

6) Copies of computer retrieved medical studies

7) Copy of changed Surgical Consent Form

8) Copy of changed Hospital Admission Form

9) Doctor's agreement to waive excessive fees

10) Copy of Living Will

It is possible that "getting it in writing" may be your best action for assuring the quality of your healthcare treatment. The healthcare industry has done a very poor job of giving patient information, while having the patient sign forms that state the patient doesn't want information. This is your way of saying I want information and I want it in writing; don't hide information from me.

"SMARTER" CONSUMER HABITS

(Traditional Patient)	(Informed Patient)
Feel Ill	Feel Ill Use Home Medical Library Dr. Visit Required Qualify Dr. Prepare History
Visit Dr. History Taken Exam	Visit Dr. History Taken Exam
Diagnostic Testing (Opt.)	Qualify Lab Cost Estimate Benefits/Risk Diagnostic Testing
Report of Findings	Report of Findings Treatment Research Support Groups Data Base Medical Library Risk Assessment Cost Estimate
Treatment (Office)	Treatment (Office)
Specialist Referral (Opt.)	Qualify Specialist Specialist Referral (Opt.)
Hospitalization (Opt.)	Qualify Hospital Cost Estimate Risk Assessment Hospitalization

WORDS OR PHRASES
TO HELP GET YOU STARTED

Here are a few key words and phrases to help you start a dialogue with your doctor. It is important to use non-adversarial words as you want information to make an informed medical treatment decision.

Start Any Discussion — "Tell me about . . ."

Doctor References — "Maybe one or two of your patients would talk to me if you would call them."

About Price — "How much?"
"How about a copy of a previous bill?"
"You mean I don't have to pay anything?"
"Will you waive excess?"

Doctor Referrals — "Please give me the name of three doctors so I can choose the one with which I would be most comfortable."

Treatment Risk — "What else can go wrong?"

Surgical Consent Form/Risk Assessment — "But isn't this what we discussed?"

Understanding — "I'm having trouble understanding you, could you put it in simpler terms. I can't agree to anything I don't understand. Can you give me something to read at my leisure?"

Hospital Complication Rates — "It is probably available in your medical malpractice loss run."

Hospital Infection Rates — "It is probably available in your JCAHO infection control report."

Hospital Mortality Rates — "It is probably available in your HCFA report."

. . . to be continued

APPENDIX A

AMA Ethics and Current Opinions

Author's Brief Index

CONTENTS

AMERICAN MEDICAL ASSOCIATION
PRINCIPLES OF MEDICAL ETHICS

PREAMBLE:

The medical profession has long subscribed to a body of ethical statements developed primarily for the benefit of the patient. As a member of this profession, a physician must recognize responsibility not only to patients, but also to society, to other health professionals, and to self. The following Principles adopted by the American Medical Association are not laws, but standards of conduct which define the essentials of honorable behavior for the physician.

I.   A physician shall be dedicated to providing competent medical service with compassion and respect for human dignity.

II.   A physician shall deal honestly with patients and colleagues, and strive to expose those physicians deficient in character or competence, or who engage in fraud or deception.

III. A physician shall respect the law and also recognize a responsibility to seek changes in those requirements which are contrary to the best interests of the patient.

IV.   A physician shall respect the rights of patients, of colleagues, and of other health professionals, and shall safeguard patient confidences within the constraints of the law.

V.   A physician shall continue to study, apply and advance scientific knowledge, make relevant information available to patients, colleagues, and the public, obtain consultation, and use the talents of other health professionals when indicated.

VI.   A physician shall, in the provision of appropriate patient care, except in emergencies, be free to choose whom to serve, with whom to associate, and the environment in which to provide medical services.

VII. A physician shall recognize a responsibility to participate in activities contributing to an improved community.

1.00   INTRODUCTION

1.01   TERMINOLOGY. Historically, the term "ethical" has been used in opinions of the Council on Ethical and Judicial Affairs and in resolutions adopted by the House of Delegates to refer to matters involving (1) moral principles or practices; (2) customs and usages of the medical profession; and (3) matters of policy not necessarily involving issues of morality in the practice of medicine. The term "unethical" has been used to refer to conduct which fails to conform to these professional standards, customs and usages, or policies.

Unethical conduct involving moral principles, values and duties calls for disciplinary action such as censure, suspension, or expulsion from medical society membership.

Failure to conform to the customs and usages of the medical profession may call for disciplinary action depending upon the particular circumstances involved, local attitudes, and how the conduct in question may reflect upon the dignity of and respect for the medical profession.

In matters strictly of a policy nature, a physician who disagrees with the position of the American Medical Association is entitled to freedom and protection of his point of view.

1.02   THE RELATION OF LAW AND ETHICS. The following statements are intended to clarify the interrelationship between law and ethics.

Ethical standards of professional conduct and responsibility may exceed but are never less than, nor contrary to, those required by law.

Violation of governmental laws may subject the physician to civil or criminal liability. Expulsion from membership is the maximum penalty that may be imposed by a medical society upon a physician who violates the ethical standards involving a breach of moral duty or principle. However, medical societies have a civic and professional obligation to report to the appropriate governmental body or state board of medical examiners credible evidence that may come to their attention involving the alleged criminal conduct of any physician relating to the practice of medicine.

Although a physician charged with allegedly illegal conduct may be acquitted or exonerated in civil or criminal proceedings, this does not discharge a medical society from its obligation to initiate a disciplinary proceeding against a member with reference to the same conduct where there is credible evidence tending to establish unethical conduct.

Ethical pronouncements of the Council on Ethical and Judicial Affairs and the House of Delegates should not be so interpreted, construed or applied as to encourage conduct which violates a valid law.

2.00   OPINIONS ON SOCIAL POLICY ISSUES

2.01   ABORTION. The Principles of Medical Ethics of the AMA do not prohibit a physician from performing an abortion in accordance with good medical practice and under circumstances that do not violate the law. (IV)

2.02   ABUSE OF CHILDREN, ELDERLY PERSONS, AND OTHERS AT RISK. Laws that require the reporting of cases of suspected abuse of children and elderly persons often create a difficult dilemma for the physician. The parties involved, both the suspected offenders and the victims, will often plead with the physician that the matter be kept confidential and not be disclosed or reported for investigation by public authorities.

Children who have been seriously injured, apparently by their parents, may nevertheless try to protect their parents by saying that the injuries were caused by an accident, such as a fall. The reason may stem from the natural parent-child relationship or fear of further punishment. Even institutionalized elderly patients who have been physically maltreated may be concerned that disclosure of what has occurred might lead to further and more drastic maltreatment by those responsible.

The physician who fails to comply with the laws requiring reporting of suspected cases of abuse to children and elderly persons and others at risk can expect that the victims could receive more severe abuse that may result in permanent bodily or brain injury or even death.

Public officials concerned with the welfare of children and elderly persons have expressed the opinion that the incidence of physical violence to these persons is rapidly increasing and that a very substantial percentage of such cases is unreported by hospital personnel and physicians. An important element that is sometimes overlooked is that a child or elderly person brought to a physician with a suspicious injury is the patient whose interests require the protection of law in a particular situation, even though the physician may also provide services from time to time to parents or other members of the family.

The obligation to comply with statutory requirements is clearly stated in the Principles of Medical Ethics. As stated at 1.02, the ethical obligation of the physician may exceed the statutory legal requirement. (I,III)

2.03 **ALLOCATION OF HEALTH RESOURCES.** A physician has a duty to do all that he can for the benefit of his individual patient. To expect a physician when treating a patient to make rationing decisions based on governmental or other external priorities in the allocation of scarce health resources creates an undesirable conflict with the primary responsibility of the physician to his patient.

Societal decisions regarding the allocation of limited health care resources should be based on fair, socially acceptable, and humane criteria. Priority should be given to persons who are most likely to be treated successfully or derive long term benefit. Utility or relative worth to society must not determine whether an individual is accepted as a donor or recipient for transplantation, selected for human experimentation, or denied or given preference in receiving costly or scarce health care therapy or resources.

Physicians as citizens have a responsibility to participate and to contribute their professional expertise in decisions made at the societal level regarding the allocation or rationing of health resources. (I,VII)

2.04 **ARTIFICIAL INSEMINATION.** The informed consent of the woman seeking artificial insemination and her husband is necessary. The prospective parents should be informed that any child conceived by artificial insemination is possessed of and entitled to all the rights of a child conceived naturally. (I,V)

2.05 **ARTIFICIAL INSEMINATION BY DONOR.** Physicians have an ethical responsibility to use the utmost caution and scientifically available screening techniques in the selection of donors for use in artificial insemination. Relying only upon the verbal representations of donors as to their health, without any medical screening, is precarious. The donor should be screened for genetic defects, inheritable and infectious disease, Rh factor incompatibility and other disorders that may affect the fetus. When the physician is not equipped to fulfill these responsibilities, the services of a skilled medical geneticist or other appropriate specialist should be sought.

Since the identity of donors usually should not be available to recipients or the offspring that may result, the risk of inadvertent inbred and serious undesirable genetic and biological consequences should not be ignored. Physicians have an ethical and social responsibility to avoid the frequent use of semen from the same sources. (I,V)

2.06 **CAPITAL PUNISHMENT.** An individual's opinion on capital punishment is the personal moral decision of the individual. A physician, as a member of a profession dedicated to preserving life when there is hope of doing so, should not be a participant in a legally authorized execution. A physician may make a determination or certification of death as currently provided by law in any situation. (I)

2.07   **CLINICAL INVESTIGATION.** The following guidelines are intended to aid physicians in fulfilling their ethical responsibilities when they engage in the clinical investigation of new drugs and procedures.

(1) A physician may participate in clinical investigation only to the extent that those activities are a part of a systematic program competently designed, under accepted standards of scientific research, to produce data which are scientifically valid and significant.

(2) In conducting clinical investigation, the investigator should demonstrate the same concern and caution for the welfare, safety, and comfort of the person involved as is required of a physician who is furnishing medical care to a patient independent of any clinical investigation.

(3) In clinical investigation primarily for treatment—

    A. The physician must recognize that the physician-patient relationship exists and that professional judgment and skill must be exercised in the best interest of the patient.

    B. Voluntary written consent must be obtained from the patient, or from his legally authorized representative if the patient lacks the capacity to consent, following: (a) disclosure that the physician intends to use an investigational drug or experimental procedure, (b) a reasonable explanation of the nature of the drug or procedure to be used, risks to be expected, and possible therapeutic benefits, (c) an offer to answer any inquiries concerning the drug or procedure, and (d) a disclosure of alternative drugs or procedures that may be available.

        i. In exceptional circumstances and to the extent that disclosure of information concerning the nature of the drug or experimental procedure or risks would be expected to materially affect the health of the patient and would be detrimental to his best interests, such information may be withheld from the patient. In such circumstances, such information shall be disclosed to a responsible relative or friend of the patient where possible.

        ii. Ordinarily, consent should be in writing, except where the physician deems it necessary to rely upon consent in other than written form because of the physical or emotional state of the patient.

        iii. Where emergency treatment is necessary, the patient is incapable of giving consent, and no one is available who has authority to act on his behalf, consent is assumed.

(4) In clinical investigation primarily for the accumulation of scientific knowledge—

    A. Adequate safeguards must be provided for the welfare, safety and comfort of the subject. It is fundamental social policy that the advancement of scientific knowledge must always be secondary to primary concern for the individual.

    B. Consent, in writing, should be obtained from the subject, or from his legally authorized representative if the subject lacks the capacity to consent, following: (a) a disclosure of the fact that an investigational drug or procedure is to be used, (b) a reasonable explanation of the nature of the procedure to be used and risks to be expected, and (c) an offer to answer any inquiries concerning the drug or procedure.

    C. Minors or mentally incompetent persons may be used as subjects only if:

        i. The nature of the investigation is such that mentally competent adults would not be suitable subjects.

       ii. Consent, in writing, is given by a legally authorized representative of the subject under circumstances in which an informed and prudent adult would reasonably be expected to volunteer himself or his child as a subject.

    D. No person may be used as a subject against his will.

    E. The overuse of institutionalized persons in research is an unfair distribution of research risks. Participation is coercive and not voluntary if the participant is subjected to powerful incentives and persuasion. (I,III,V)

2.08   **CLINICAL INVESTIGATION: REPLACEMENT OF VITAL HUMAN ORGANS.** The following are guidelines, suggested by the Council, in conducting experimental or clinical investigation, such as with mechanical devices or animal organs, for the replacement of human organs that are no longer functional:

    (1) Experimental or clinical investigations should be conducted as part of a systematic program competently designed, under accepted standards of scientific research, to produce data which are scientifically valid and significant.

    (2) The physicians conducting clinical investigations should demonstrate the same concern and caution for the welfare, safety, and comfort of the persons involved as is required of physicians who are furnishing medical care to patients independent of any clinical investigation.

    (3) Voluntary written consent must be obtained from the patient, or from his legally authorized representative if the patient lacks capacity to consent, following (a) disclosure that the physician(s) intend to use an investigational or experimental procedure, (b) a reasonable explanation of the nature of the procedure to be used, risks to be expected, and possible therapeutic benefits, (c) an offer to answer any inquiries concerning the procedure, and (d) a disclosure of alternative procedures, if any, that may be available. Physicians should be completely objective in discussing the details of the procedure to be performed, the pain and discomfort that may be anticipated, known risks and possible

hazards, the quality of life to be expected, and particularly the alternatives. Especially, physicians should not use persuasion to obtain consents which otherwise might not be forthcoming, nor should expectations be encouraged beyond those which the circumstances reasonably and realistically justify.

(4) In clinical investigation primarily for the accumulation of scientific knowledge, adequate safeguards should be provided for the welfare, safety and comfort of the patient. The medical profession recognizes as fundamental social policy that the advancement of scientific knowledge must always be secondary to primary concern for the individual. The physician must never deny the patient the best possible therapeutic modality in favor of an experimental treatment which is less likely to succeed.

(5) With the approval of the patient or the patient's lawful representative, physicians should cooperate with the press and media to ensure that medical news concerning the progress of clinical investigation or the patient's condition is available more promptly and more accurately than would be possible without their assistance. On the other hand, the Council does not approve of practices designed to create fanfare, sensationalism to attract media attention, and unwarranted expressions of optimism because of short term progress, even though longer range prognosis is known from the beginning to be precarious. With the approval of the patient or the patient's family, the Council, however, encourages the objective disclosure to the press and media of pertinent information. The situation should not be used for the commercial ends of participating physicians or the institutions involved.

The Council has not evaluated nor does it have sufficient information upon which to base an evaluation as to the extent to which cases involving the use of animal organs and mechanical hearts conform to the above guidelines. These guidelines are provided to the public, the medical profession, and the scientific community in the belief that they may find them helpful in making their own independent judgments. (I,III,V)

2.09   COSTS. While physicians should be conscious of costs and not provide or prescribe unnecessary services or ancillary facilities, social policy expects that concern for the care the patient receives will be the physician's first consideration. This does not preclude the physician, individually, or through medical organizations, from participating in policy-making with respect to social issues affecting health care. (I,VII)

2.10 **FETAL RESEARCH GUIDELINES.** The following guidelines are offered as aids to physicians when they are engaged in fetal research:

(1) Physicians may participate in fetal research when their activities are part of a competently designed program, under accepted standards of scientific research, to produce data which are scientifically valid and significant.

(2) If appropriate, properly performed clinical studies on animals and nongravid humans should precede any particular fetal research project.

(3) In fetal research projects, the investigator should demonstrate the same care and concern for the fetus as a physician providing fetal care or treatment in a non-research setting.

(4) All valid federal or state legal requirements should be followed.

(5) There should be no monetary payment to obtain any fetal material for fetal research projects.

(6) Competent peer review committees, review boards, or advisory boards should be available, when appropriate, to protect against the possible abuses that could arise in such research.

(7) Research on the so called "dead fetus," mascerated fetal material, fetal cells, fetal tissue, or fetal organs should be in accord with state laws on autopsy and state laws on organ transplantation or anatomical gifts.

(8) In fetal research primarily for treatment of the fetus:

    A. Voluntary and informed consent, in writing, should be given by the gravid woman, acting in the best interest of the fetus.

    B. Alternative treatment or methods of care, if any, should be carefully evaluated and fully explained. If simpler and safer treatment is available, it should be pursued.

(9) In research primarily for treatment of the gravid female:

    A. Voluntary and informed consent, in writing, should be given by the patient.

    B. Alternative treatment or methods of care should be carefully evaluated and fully explained to the patient. If simpler and safer treatment is available, it should be pursued.

    C. If possible, the risk to the fetus should be the least possible, consistent with the gravid female's need for treatment.

(10) In fetal research involving a viable fetus, primarily for the accumulation of scientific knowledge:

    A. Voluntary and informed consent, in writing, should be given by the gravid woman under circumstances in which a prudent and informed adult would reasonably be expected to give such consent.

    B. The risk to the fetus imposed by the research should be the least possible.

C. The purpose of research is the production of data and knowledge which are scientifically significant and which cannot otherwise be obtained.

D. In this area of research, it is especially important to emphasize that care and concern for the fetus should be demonstrated. There should be no physical abuse of the fetus. (I,III,V)

2.11   **GENE THERAPY.** Gene therapy involves the insertion of a normally functioning gene into cells in which an abnormal or absent element of the gene has caused disease, with the goal of restoring normal cellular function. The replacement gene may be inserted into target cells either in situ or outside the body for later reimplantation.

Two types of gene therapy have been identified: (1) somatic cell therapy, in which human cells other than germ cells are genetically altered, and (2) germ line therapy, in which a replacement gene is integrated into the genome of human gametes or their precursors, resulting in expression of the new gene in the patient's offspring and subsequent generations. The fundamental difference between germ line therapy and somatic cell therapy is that germ line therapy affects the welfare of subsequent generations and may be associated with increased risk and the potential for unpredictable and irreversible results.

The goal of both somatic and germ line therapy is to alleviate human suffering and disease by remedying disorders for which available therapies are not satisfactory. This goal should be pursued only within the ethical tradition of medicine, which gives primacy to the welfare of the patient whose safety and well-being must be vigorously protected. To the extent possible, experience with animal studies must be sufficient to assure the effectiveness and safety of the techniques used, and the predictability of the results.

Moreover, gene therapy should be utilized only for therapeutic purposes. Efforts to enhance "desirable" characteristics through the insertion of a modified or additional gene, or efforts to "improve" complex human traits—the eugenic development of offspring—are contrary not only to the ethical tradition of medicine, but also to the egalitarian values of our society and should not be pursued.

In summary, somatic cell and germ line therapy should:

(1) conform to the Council on Ethical and Judicial Affairs' guidelines on clinical investigation and genetic engineering;

(2) adhere to stringent safety considerations; and

(3) be utilized only for therapeutic purposes in the treatment of human disorders—not for the enhancement or eugenic development of patients or their offspring. (I,V)

2.12   **GENETIC COUNSELING.** Two primary areas of genetic diagnosis are: (1) screening or evaluating prospective parents before conception for genetic disease to predict the likelihood of conceiving an affected child; and (2) in utero testing after conception, such as ultrasonography, amniocentesis, and fetoscopy, to determine the condition of the fetus. Physicians engaged in genetic counseling are ethically obligated to provide prospective parents with the basis for an informed decision for childbearing. In providing information to couples who choose to reproduce, physicians should adhere to the Principles of Medical Ethics and standards of medical practice.

Technological developments in the accuracy of predicting and detecting genetic disorders have created a dilemma for the physician who for personal reasons opposes contraception, sterilization or abortion. The physician should be aware that where a genetic defect is found in the fetus, prospective parents may request or refuse an abortion. A dilemma may also exist for physicians who do not oppose the provision of these services (contraception, sterilization or abortion).

Physicians who consider the legal and ethical requirements applicable to genetic counseling to be in conflict with their moral values and conscience may choose to limit such services to preconception diagnosis and advice or not provide any genetic services. However, there are circumstances in which the physician who is so disposed is nevertheless obligated to alert prospective parents that a potential genetic problem does exist, that the physician does not offer genetic services, and that the patient should seek medical genetic counseling from another qualified specialist.

Physicians, whether they oppose or do not oppose contraception, sterilization or abortion, may decide that they can engage in **gene**tic counseling and screening but should avoid the imposition of their personal moral values and the substitution of their own moral judgment for that of the prospective parents. (II,IV,V,VI)

2.13   **GENETIC ENGINEERING.** Whatever form of regulation of gene splicing, recombinant DNA research, chemical synthesis of DNA molecules, or other genetic engineering research is eventually developed, there should be independent input from the scientific community, organized medicine, industry, and others, in addition to the federal government, to prevent abuse from any sector of society, private or public.

If and when gene replacement with normal DNA becomes a practical reality for the treatment of human disorders, the following factors should be considered:

(1) If procedures are performed in a research setting, reference should be made to the Council's guidelines on clinical investigation.

(2) If procedures are performed in a non-research setting, adherence to usual and customary standards of medical practice and professional responsibility would be required.

(3) Full discussion of the proposed procedure with the patient would be required. The consent of the patient or his legal representative should be informed, voluntary and written.

(4) There must be no hazardous or other unwanted virus on the viral DNA containing the replacement or corrective gene.

(5) The inserted DNA must function under normal control within the recipient cell to prevent metabolic damage that could damage tissue and the patient.

(6) The effectiveness of the gene therapy should be evaluated as best as possible. This will include determination of the natural history of the disease and follow-up examination of subsequent generations.

(7) Such procedures should be undertaken in the future only after careful evaluation of the availability and effectiveness of other possible therapy. If simpler and safer treatment is available, it should be pursued.

(8) These considerations should be reviewed, as appropriate, as procedures and scientific information are developed in the future. (I,V,VII)

2.14   IN VITRO FERTILIZATION. The technique of in vitro fertilization and embryo transplantation enables certain couples previously incapable of conception to bear a child. It is also useful in the field of research directed toward an understanding of how genetic defects arise and are transmitted and how they might be prevented or treated. Because of serious ethical and moral concerns, however, any fertilized egg that has the potential for human life and that will be implanted in the uterus of a woman should not be subjected to laboratory research.

All fertilized ova not utilized for implantation and that are maintained for research purposes shall be handled with the strictest adherence to the Principles of Medical Ethics, to the guidelines for research and medical practice expressed in the Council's opinion on fetal research, and to the highest standards of medical practice. (I,IV,V)

2.15   ORGAN DONATION. The voluntary donation of organs in appropriate circumstances is to be encouraged. However, it is not ethical to participate in a procedure to enable a donor to receive payment, other than for the reimbursement of expenses necessarily incurred in connection with removal, for any of the donor's non-renewable organs. (I,III,V)

2.16   **ORGAN TRANSPLANTATION GUIDELINES.** The following statement is offered for guidance of physicians as they seek to maintain the highest level of ethical conduct in the transplanting of human organs.

(1) In all professional relationships between a physician and his patient, the physician's primary concern must be the health of his patient. He owes the patient his primary allegiance. This concern and allegiance must be preserved in all medical procedures, including those which involve the transplantation of an organ from one person to another where both donor and recipient are patients. Care must, therefore, be taken to protect the rights of both the donor and the recipient, and no physician may assume a responsibility in organ transplantation unless the rights of both donor and recipient are equally protected.

(2) A prospective organ transplant offers no justification for a relaxation of the usual standard of medical care. The physician should provide his patient, who may be a prospective organ donor, with that care usually given others being treated for a similar injury or disease.

(3) When a vital, single organ is to be transplanted, the death of the donor shall have been determined by at least one physician other than the recipient's physician. Death shall be determined by the clinical judgment of the physician. In making this determination, the ethical physician will use currently accepted and available scientific tests.

(4) Full discussion of the proposed procedure with the donor and the recipient or their responsible relatives or representatives is mandatory. The physician should be objective in discussing the procedure, in disclosing known risks and possible hazards, and in advising of the alternative procedures available. The physician should not encourage expectations beyond those which the circumstances justify. The physician's interest in advancing scientific knowledge must always be secondary to his primary concern for the patient.

(5) Transplant procedures of body organs should be undertaken (a) only by physicians who possess special medical knowledge and technical competence developed through special training, study, and laboratory experience and practice, and (b) in medical institutions with facilities adequate to protect the health and well-being of the parties to the procedure.

(6) Transplantation of body organs should be undertaken only after careful evaluation of the availability and effectiveness of other possible therapy. (I,III,V)

2.17   **QUALITY OF LIFE.** In the making of decisions for the treatment of seriously deformed newborns or persons who are severely deteriorated victims of injury, illness or advanced age, the primary consideration should be what is best for the individual patient and not the avoidance of a burden to the family or to society. Quality of life is a factor to be considered in determining what is best for the individual. Life should be cherished despite disabilities and handicaps, except when the prolongation would be inhumane and unconscionable. Under these circumstances, withholding or removing life supporting means is ethical provided that the normal care given an individual who is ill is not discontinued. (I,III,IV)

2.18   **SURROGATE MOTHERS.** "Surrogate" motherhood is an arrangement which involves the artificial insemination of a woman who agrees to give the child, thus conceived, for adoption by the man providing the semen and, usually, his infertile wife. The arrangement involves the services of an attorney who attends to the legal phases of the transaction, a physician who will perform or arrange for the medical services that may be required, and the person or persons seeking a child for adoption. A woman is sought to enter into a contract to bear a child and surrender that child for adoption. The contract customarily provides compensation for costs of the medical services and for living expenses of the surrogate mother during pregnancy, as well as for discomfort or inconvenience.

The Council is concerned about the ethical, social and legal problems that may arise in an arrangement in which a woman agrees to become pregnant through artificial insemination, to carry to term and to give the child thus conceived to other persons to serve as adoptive parents. The welfare of the child should be a foremost consideration. In ordinary adoption proceedings an appropriate agency usually investigates prospective parents to determine their fitness as parents. This precaution is not always present in surrogate motherhood arrangements.

The Council is also concerned that, if there is a subsequent birth of a defective child, a situation may arise in which prospective adoptive parents and the woman who gave birth to the child may not want to or will be unable to assume the responsibilities of parenthood.

Many other ethical, social and morally difficult situations can be envisioned. For example, the woman who has contracted to bear the child may decide to have an abortion or to refuse to give the child up for adoption. Another consideration which may be overlooked is the psychological impairment that may occur in a woman who deliberately conceives with the intention of bearing a child which she will give up.

The Council believes that surrogate motherhood does not represent a satisfactory reproductive alternative for people who wish to become parents because of the many associated ethical, legal, psychological, societal, and financial concerns. (I,II,IV)

2.19   **UNNECESSARY SERVICES.** Physicians should not provide, prescribe, or seek compensation for services that are known to be unnecessary or worthless. (II,VII)

2.20   **WITHHOLDING OR WITHDRAWING LIFE-PROLONGING MEDICAL TREATMENT.** The social commitment of the physician is to sustain life and relieve suffering. Where the performance of one duty conflicts with the other, the preferences of the patient should prevail. If the patient is incompetent to act in his own behalf and did not previously indicate his preferences, the family or other surrogate decisionmaker, in concert with the physician, must act in the best interest of the patient.

For humane reasons, with informed consent, a physician may do what is medically necessary to alleviate severe pain, or cease or omit treatment to permit a terminally ill patient to die when death is imminent. However, the physician should not intentionally cause death. In deciding whether the administration of potentially life-prolonging medical treatment is in the best interest of the patient who is incompetent to act in his own behalf, the surrogate decisionmaker and physician should consider several factors, including: the possibility for extending life under humane and comfortable conditions; the patient's values about life and the way it should be lived; and the patient's attitudes toward sickness, suffering, medical procedures, and death.

Even if death is not imminent but a patient is beyond doubt permanently unconscious, and there are adequate safeguards to confirm the accuracy of the diagnosis, it is not unethical to discontinue all means of life-prolonging medical treatment.

Life-prolonging medical treatment includes medication and artificially or technologically supplied respiration, nutrition or hydration. In treating a terminally ill or permanently unconscious patient, the dignity of the patient should be maintained at all times. (I,III,IV,V)

2.21   **WITHHOLDING OR WITHDRAWING LIFE-PROLONGING MEDICAL TREATMENT-PATIENTS' PREFERENCES.** A competent, adult patient may, in advance, formulate and provide a valid consent to the withholding or withdrawal of life-support systems in the event that injury or illness renders that individual incompetent to make such a decision. The preference of the individual should prevail when determining whether extraordinary life-prolonging measures should be undertaken in the event of terminal illness. Unless it is clearly established that the patient is terminally ill or permanently unconscious, a physician should not be deterred from appropriately aggressive treatment of a patient. (I,III,IV,V)

3.00 OPINIONS ON INTERPROFESSIONAL RELATIONS

3.01 NONSCIENTIFIC PRACTITIONERS. It is wrong to engage in or to aid and abet in treatment which has no scientific basis and is dangerous, is calculated to deceive the patient by giving him false hope, or which may cause the patient to delay in seeking proper care until his condition becomes irreversible.

Physicians should also be mindful of state laws which prohibit a physician from aiding and abetting an unlicensed person in the practice of medicine, aiding or abetting a person with a limited license in providing services beyond the scope of his license, or undertaking the joint medical treatment of patients under the foregoing circumstances.

A physician is otherwise free to accept or decline to serve anyone who seeks his services, regardless of who has recommended that the individual see the physician. (III,VI)

3.02 NURSES. The primary bond between medical practice and nursing is mutual ethical concern for patients. One of the duties in providing reasonable care is fulfilled by a nurse who carries out the orders of the attending physician. Where orders appear to the nurse to be in error or contrary to customary medical and nursing practice, the physician has an ethical obligation to explain those orders to the nurse involved. Whenever a nurse recognizes or suspects error or discrepancy in a physician's orders, the nurse has an obligation to call this to the attention of the physician. The ethical physician should neither expect nor insist that nurses follow orders contrary to standards of good medical and nursing practice. In emergencies, when prompt action is necessary and the physician is not immediately available, in the performance of reasonable care a nurse may be justified in acting contrary to the physician's standing orders for the safety of the patient. Such occurrences should not be considered to be a breakdown in professional relations. (IV,V)

3.03 OPTOMETRY. An ophthalmologist may employ an optometrist as ancillary personnel to assist him provided the optometrist is identified to patients as an optometrist.

A physician may send his patient to a qualified and ethical optometrist for optometric services. The physician would be ethically remiss, of course, if before doing so he did not ensure that there was an absence of any medical reason for his patient's complaint, and he would be equally remiss if he sent a patient without having made a medical evaluation of the patient's condition.

Physicians may teach in recognized schools of optometry for the purpose of improving the quality of optometric education. The scope of this teaching may embrace subjects within the legitimate scope of optometry which are designed to prepare students to engage in optometry within the limits prescribed by law. (V,VI)

3.04   **REFERRAL OF PATIENTS.** A physician may refer a patient for diagnostic or therapeutic services to another physician, limited practitioner, or any other provider of health care services permitted by law to furnish such services, whenever he believes that this may benefit the patient. As in the case of referrals to physician-specialists, referrals to limited practitioners should be based on their individual competence and ability to perform the services needed by the patient. A physician should not so refer a patient unless he is confident that the services provided on referral will be performed competently and in accordance with accepted scientific standards and legal requirements. (V.VI)

3.05   **SPECIALISTS.** A physician may choose to limit his practice to a specialty or to certain specialized services. He may also choose to provide services as a consultant to patients sent to him by other physicians, or to all patients at a hospital with which he has a contractual arrangement. He may, as an independent practitioner, choose to accept or decline patients sent to him by licensed limited practitioners, by laymen, or by others.

A physician may choose those persons whom he will accept as patients and also may exercise his choice by the terms of contractual arrangements with other physicians, medical groups, hospitals or other institutions. A physician may freely choose those whom he will serve, in the absence of legal considerations to the contrary.

The obligations which a physician has to provide information to a patient or any other party are those required by customary good medical practice and law. Although a physician may choose to limit his practice to certain diagnostic services, he may not neglect a patient under his care. (V,VI)

3.06   **SPORTS MEDICINE.** The rules and conditions governing amateur and professional contact sports such as boxing, football and hockey, and the extent to which the risks of bodily injury shall be acceptable to society, require informed decision-making in which the medical profession has an essential role.

The professional responsibility of the physician who serves in a medical capacity at an athletic contest or sporting event is to protect the health and safety of the contestants. The desire of spectators, promoters of the event or even the injured athlete that he should not be removed from the contest should not be controlling. The physician's judgment should be governed only by medical considerations. (I,VII)

3.07   **TEACHING.** Physicians are free to engage in any teaching permitted by law for which they are qualified. (V,VII)

4.00 OPINIONS ON HOSPITAL RELATIONS

4.01 **ADMISSION FEE.** Charging a separate and distinct fee for the incidental, administrative, non-medical service the physician performs in securing the admission of a patient to a hospital is not in keeping with the traditions of the American Medical Association and is unethical. (IV)

4.02 **ASSESSMENTS, COMPULSORY.** It is improper to condition medical staff membership or privileges on compulsory assessments for any purpose. (IV)

4.03 **BILLING FOR HOUSESTAFF SERVICES.** When a physician assumes responsibility for the services rendered to a **patient** by a resident, the physician may ethically bill the patient for services which were performed under the physician's personal observation, direction and supervision. (II)

4.04 **ECONOMIC INCENTIVES AND LEVELS OF CARE.** The primary obligation of the hospital medical staff is to safeguard the quality of care provided within the institution. The medical staff has the responsibility to perform essential functions on behalf of the hospital in accordance with licensing laws and accreditation requirements. Treatment or hospitalization that is willfully excessive or inadequate constitutes unethical practice. The organized medical staff has an obligation to avoid wasteful practices and unnecessary treatment that may cause the hospital needless expense. In a situation where the economic interests of the hospital are in conflict with patient welfare, patient welfare takes priority. (I,II,IV,V,VI)

4.05 **ORGANIZED MEDICAL STAFF.** The organized medical staff is an integral part of the hospital structure. Under authority delegated by the governing board, it performs essential hospital functions. The organized medical staff conducts professional activities that are designed to improve professional skills and to enhance the quality of patient care in the hospital.

The organized medical staff performs essential hospital functions even though it may often consist primarily of independent practicing physicians who are not hospital employees. As a practical matter, however, the organized medical staff may enjoy a dual status. In addition to functioning as a division of the hospital, members of the organized medical staff may choose to act as a group for the purpose of communicating and dealing with the governing board and others with respect to matters that concern the interest of the organized medical staff and its members. This is ethical so long as there is no adverse interference with patient care or violation of applicable laws. (IV,VI)

4.06 **PHYSICIAN-HOSPITAL CONTRACTUAL RELATIONS.** There are various financial or contractual arrangements that physicians and hospitals may enter into and find mutually satisfactory. A physician may, for example, be a hospital employee, a hospital-associated medical specialist, or an independent practitioner with staff privileges. The form of the contractual or financial arrangement between physicians and hospitals depends on the facts and circumstances of each situation. A physician may be employed by a hospital for a fixed annual amount, for a certain amount per hour, or pursuant to other similar arrangements that are related to the professional services, skill, education, expertise, or time involved.

Any conduct that results in the provision of unnecessary services or overutilization of services or facilities is, of course, unethical and should be discouraged. If such problems arise, though, these problems should be addressed directly and considered in the light of the facts and circumstances of the particular situation. (VI)

4.07 **STAFF PRIVILEGES.** The mutual objective of both the governing board and the medical staff is to improve the quality and efficiency of patient care in the hospital. Decisions regarding hospital privileges should be based upon the training, experience and demonstrated competence of candidates, taking into consideration the availability of facilities and the overall medical needs of the community, the hospital and especially patients. Personal friendships, antagonisms, jurisdictional disputes or fear of competition should be disregarded in making these decisions. Physicians who are involved in the granting, denying or termination of hospital privileges have an ethical responsibility to be guided primarily by concern for the welfare and best interests of patients in discharging this responsibility. (IV,VI,VII)

5.00 OPINIONS ON CONFIDENTIALITY, ADVERTISING AND COMMUNICATIONS MEDIA RELATIONS

5.01   ADVERTISING AND HMOs. A physician may provide medical services to members of a prepaid medical care plan or to members of a health maintenance organization which seeks members or subscribers through advertising. Physicians practicing in prepaid plans or HMO's are subject to the same ethical principles as are other physicians. Advertising which would lead prospective members or subscribers to believe that the services of a named physician who has a reputation for outstanding skill would be routinely available to all members or subscribers, if in fact this is not so, is deceptive. However, the publication by name of the roster of physicians who provide services to members, the type of practice in which each is engaged, biographical and other relevant information is not a deceptive practice. (II,VI)

5.02   ADVERTISING AND PUBLICITY. There are no restrictions on advertising by physicians except those that can be specifically justified to protect the public from deceptive practices. A physician may publicize himself as a physician through any commercial publicity or other form of public communication (including any newspaper, magazine, telephone, directory, radio, television, direct mail or other advertising) provided that the communication shall not be misleading because of the omission of necessary material information, shall not contain any false or misleading statement, or shall not otherwise operate to deceive.

Because the public can sometimes be deceived by the use of medical terms or illustrations that are difficult to understand, physicians should design the form of communication to communicate the information contained therein to the public in a readily comprehensible manner. Aggressive, high pressure advertising and publicity should be avoided if they create unjustified medical expectations or are accompanied by deceptive claims. The key issue, however, is whether advertising or publicity, regardless of format or content, is true and not materially misleading.

The communication may include: (a) the educational background of the physician; (b) the basis on which fees are determined (including charges for specific services); (c) available credit or other methods of payment; and (d) any other nondeceptive information.

Nothing in this opinion is intended to discourage or to limit advertising and representations which are not false or deceptive within the meaning of Section 5 of the Federal Trade Commission Act. At the same time, however, physicians are advised that certain types of communications have a significant potential for deception and should therefore receive special attention. For example, testimonials of patients as to the physician's skill or the quality of his professional services tend to be deceptive when they do not reflect the results that patients with conditions comparable to the testimoniant's condition generally receive.

Statements relating to the quality of medical services can raise concerns because they are extremely difficult, if not impossible, to verify or measure by objective standards. However, objective claims regarding experience, competence and the quality of the physician's services may be made if they are factually supportable. Similarly, generalized statements of satisfaction with a physician's services may be made if they are representative of the experiences of that physician's patients.

Because physicians have an ethical obligation to share medical advances, it is unlikely that a physician will have a truly exclusive or unique skill or remedy. Claims that imply such a skill or remedy therefore can be deceptive. Statements that a physician has an exclusive or unique skill or remedy in a particular geographic area, if true, however, are permissible. Similarly, a statement that a physician has cured or successfully treated a large number of cases involving a particular serious ailment is deceptive if it implies a certainty of result and creates unjustified and misleading expectations in prospective patients.

Consistent with Federal regulatory standards which apply to commercial advertising, a physician who is considering the placement of an advertisement or publicity release, whether in print, radio or television, should determine in advance that his communication or message is explicitly and implicitly truthful and not misleading. These standards require the advertiser to have a reasonable basis for claims before they are used in advertising. The reasonable basis must be established by those facts known to the advertiser, and those which a reasonable, prudent advertiser should have discovered. Inclusion of the physician's name in advertising may help to assure that these guidelines are being met. (II)

5.03   **COMMUNICATIONS MEDIA: PRESS RELATIONS.** A physician should not discuss a patient's medical condition, disease or illness with the press without the patient's authorization. The patient or the patient's lawful representative may authorize a physician to disclose health information concerning the patient to the press. The physician may release only authorized information or that which is public knowledge. (IV)

5.04   COMMUNICATIONS MEDIA: STANDARDS OF PROFESSIONAL RESPONSIBILITY. Because
certain news is a part of the public record or is a matter of concern to civil
authorities, it is readily available for publication. Physicians should cooperate
with the press to insure that medical news of this sort is available more
promptly and more accurately than would be possible without their assistance. News in this category, known as news in the public domain, includes:
births, deaths, accidents, and police cases.

The following information in the public domain can be made available
without the patient's consent:

A. Personal information: patient's name, address, age, sex, race, marital
    status, employer, occupation, name of parents in case of births,
    name of next-of-kin in case of deaths.

B. Nature of accident: Only general information regarding injuries will
    be released. This consists of the name of the injured portion of the
    body, such as back injury and the like. It may be stated that there are
    internal injuries.

    If the patient is unconscious when brought to the hospital, a
    statement to that effect may be made.

    Statements regarding the circumstances surrounding shootings,
    knifings, and poisonings are properly police matters, and questions
    whether they were accidental or otherwise should be referred to the
    appropriate authorities.

    A statement may be made to the effect that the patient was
    injured by a knife or other sharp instrument, but no statement may
    be made as to whether or not it was assault, accident, or self-inflicted.

    A statement may be made to the effect that the patient received
    burns and the member of the body affected may be indicated.

    No statement may be made that there was a suicide or attempted
    suicide.

    No statement may be made to the effect that intoxication or
    drug addiction was involved.

    No statement may be made that moral turpitude was involved.

C. Diagnosis and prognosis: Inasmuch as a diagnosis may be made only
    by a physician and may depend upon X-ray and laboratory studies,
    no statement regarding diagnosis should be made except by or on
    behalf of the attending physician. For the same reason, prognosis
    will be given only by the attending physician or at his direction.

D. Patient's condition: A statement may be made as to the general
    condition of the patient using the following classifications: minor
    injuries or similar general diagnosis, good, fair, serious, critical.

When information concerning a specific patient is requested, the
physician must obtain the consent of the patient or his authorized representative before releasing such information. The patient's decision is final under

the law. Physicians are ethically and legally required to protect the personal privacy and other legal rights of patients. The physician-patient relationship and its confidential nature must be maintained. With these considerations in mind, the physician may assist the representatives of the media in every way possible. (IV)

5.05   **CONFIDENTIALITY.** The information disclosed to a physician during the course of the relationship between physician and patient is confidential to the greatest possible degree. The patient should feel free to make a full disclosure of information to the physician in order that the physician may most effectively provide needed services. The patient should be able to make this disclosure with the knowledge that the physician will respect the confidential nature of the communication. The physician should not reveal confidential communications or information without the express consent of the patient, unless required to do so by law.

    The obligation to safeguard patient confidences is subject to certain exceptions which are ethically and legally justified because of overriding social considerations. Where a patient threatens to inflict serious bodily harm to another person and there is a reasonable probability that the patient may carry out the threat, the physician should take reasonable precautions for the protection of the intended victim, including notification of law enforcement authorities. Also, communicable diseases, gun shot and knife wounds, should be reported as required by applicable statutes or ordinances. (IV)

5.06   **CONFIDENTIALITY: ATTORNEY-PHYSICIAN RELATION.** The patient's history, diagnosis, treatment, and prognosis may be discussed with the patient's lawyer with the consent of the patient or the patient's lawful representative.

    A physician may testify in court or before a workmen's compensation board or the like in any personal injury or related case. (IV)

5.07   **CONFIDENTIALITY: COMPUTERS.** The utmost effort and care must be taken to protect the confidentiality of all medical records. This ethical principle applies to computerized medical records as it applies to any other medical records.

    The confidentiality of physician-patient communications is desirable to assure free and open disclosure by the patient to the physician of all information needed to establish a proper diagnosis and attain the most desirable clinical outcome possible. Protecting the confidentiality of the personal and medical information in such medical records is also necessary to prevent humiliation, embarrassment, or discomfort of patients. At the same time, patients may have legitimate desires to have medical information concerning their care and treatment forwarded to others.

Both the protection of confidentiality and the appropriate release of information in records is the rightful expectation of the patient. A physician should respect the patient's expectations of confidentiality concerning medical records that involve the patient's care and treatment, but the physician should also respect the patient's authorization to provide information from the medical record to those whom the patient authorizes to inspect all or part of it for legitimate purposes.

Computer technology permits the accumulation, storage, and analysis of an unlimited quantum of medical information. The possibility of access to information is greater with a computerized data system than with information stored in the traditional written form in a physician's office. Accordingly, the guidelines below are offered to assist physicians and computer service organizations in maintaining the confidentiality of information in medical records when that information is stored in computerized data bases. It should be recognized that specific procedures adapted from application of these concepts may vary depending upon the nature of the organization processing the data as well as the appropriate and authorized use of the stored data.

Guidelines on a computerized data base:

(1) Confidential medical information entered into the computerized data base should be verified as to authenticity of source.

(2) The patient and physician should be advised about the existence of computerized data bases in which medical information concerning the patient is stored. Such information should be communicated to the physician and patient prior to the physician's release of the medical information. All individuals and organizations with some form of access to the computerized data bank, and the level of access permitted, should be specifically identified in advance.

(3) The physician and patient should be notified of the distribution of all reports reflecting identifiable patient data prior to distribution of the reports by the computer facility. There should be approval by the physician and patient prior to the release of patient-identifiable clinical and administrative data to individuals or organizations external to the medical care environment, and such information should not be released without the express permission of the physician and the patient.

(4) The dissemination of confidential medical data should be limited to only those individuals or agencies with a bona fide use for the data. Release of confidential medical information from the data base should be confined to the specific purpose for which the information is requested and limited to the specific time frame requested. All such organizations or individuals should be advised that authorized release of data to them does not authorize their further release of the data to additional individuals or organizations.

(5) Procedures for adding to or changing data on the computerized data base should indicate individuals authorized to make changes, time periods in which changes take place, and those individuals who will be informed about changes in the data from the medical records.

(6) Procedures for purging the computerized data base of archaic or inaccurate data should be established and the patient and physician should be notified before and after the data has been purged. There should be no commingling of a physician's computerized patient records with those of other computer service bureau clients. In addition, procedures should be developed to protect against inadvertent mixing of individual reports or segments thereof.

(7) The computerized medical data base should be on-line to the computer terminal only when authorized computer programs requiring the medical data are being used. Individuals and organizations external to the clinical facility should not be provided on-line access to a computerized data base containing identifiable data from medical records concerning patients.

(8) Security:

A. Stringent security procedures for entry into the immediate environment in which the computerized medical data base is stored and/or processed or for otherwise having access to confidential medical information should be developed and strictly enforced so as to prevent access to the computer facility by unauthorized personnel. Personnel audit procedures should be developed to establish a record in the event of unauthorized disclosure of medical data. A roster of past and present service bureau personnel with specified levels of access to the medical data base should be maintained. Specific administrative sanctions should exist to prevent employee breaches of confidentiality and security procedures.

B. All terminated or former employees in the data processing environment should have no access to data from the medical records concerning patients.

C. Involuntarily terminated employees working in the data processing environment in which data from medical records concerning patients are processed should immediately upon termination be removed from the computerized medical data environment.

D. Upon termination of computer service bureau services for a physician, those computer files maintained for the physician should be physically turned over to the physician, or destroyed (erased). In the event of file erasure, the computer service bureau should verify in writing to the physician that the erasure has taken place. (VI)

5.08   CONFIDENTIALITY: INSURANCE COMPANY REPRESENTATIVE. History, diagnosis, prognosis, and the like acquired during the physician-patient relationship may be disclosed to an insurance company representative only if the patient or his lawful representative has consented to the disclosure. A physician's responsibilities to his patient are not limited to the actual practice of medicine. They also include the performance of some services ancillary to the practice of medicine. These services might include certification that the patient was under the physician's care and comment on the diagnosis and therapy in the particular case. (IV)

5.09   CONFIDENTIALITY: PHYSICIANS IN INDUSTRY. Where a physician's services are limited to pre-employment physical examinations or examinations to determine if an employee who has been ill or injured is able to return to work, no physician-patient relationship exists between the physician and those individuals. Nevertheless, the information obtained by the physician as a result of such examinations is confidential and should not be communicated to a third party without the individual's prior written consent, unless it is required by law. If the individual authorized the release of medical information to an employer or a potential employer, the physician should release only that information which is reasonably relevant to the employer's decision regarding that individual's ability to perform the work required by the job.

A physician-patient relationship does exist when a physician renders treatment to an employee, even though the physician is paid by the employer. If the employee's illness or injury is work-related, the release of medical information as to the treatment provided to the employer may be subject to the provisions of workers compensation laws. The physician must comply with the requirements of such laws, if applicable. However, the physician may not otherwise discuss the employee's health condition with the employer without the employee's consent or, in the event of the employee's incapacity, the family's consent.

Whenever statistical information about employees' health is released, all employee identities should be deleted. (IV)

6.00   ## OPINIONS ON FEES AND CHARGES

6.01   **CONTINGENT PHYSICIAN FEES.** If a physician's fee for medical service is contingent on the successful outcome of a claim, there is the ever-present danger that the physician may become less of a healer and more of an advocate. Accordingly, a physician's fee for medical services should be based on the value of the service provided by the physician to the patient and not on the uncertain outcome of a contingency that does not in any way relate to the value of the medical service. (IV)

6.02   **FEE SPLITTING.** Payment by one physician to another solely for the referral of a patient is fee splitting and is improper both for the physician making the payment and the physician receiving the payment.

A physician may not accept payment of any kind, in any form, from any source, such as a pharmaceutical company or pharmacist, an optical company or the manufacturer of medical appliances and devices, for prescribing or referring a patient to said source for the purchase of drugs, glasses or appliances.

In each case, the payment violates the requirement to deal honestly with patients and colleagues. The patient relies upon the advice of the physician on matters of referral. All referrals and prescriptions must be based on the skill and quality of the physician to whom the patient has been referred or the quality and efficacy of the drug or product prescribed. (II)

6.03   **FEE SPLITTING: CLINIC OR LABORATORY REFERRALS.** Clinics or laboratories that compensate physicians based solely on the amount of work referred by the physician to the clinic or laboratory are engaged in fee splitting which is unethical. (II) [Superseded by 6.05.]

6.04   **FEE SPLITTING: DRUG OR DEVICE PRESCRIPTION REBATES.** A physician may not accept any kind of payment or compensation from a drug company or device manufacturer for prescribing its products. The physician should keep the following considerations in mind:

(1) A physician should only prescribe a drug or device based on his reasonable expectations of the effectiveness of the drug or device for the particular patient.

(2) The quantity of the drug prescribed should be no greater than that which is reasonably required for the patient's condition. (II)

6.05   **FEE SPLITTING: REFERRALS TO HEALTH CARE FACILITIES.** Clinics, laboratories, hospitals, or other health care facilities that compensate physicians based solely on the amount of work referred by the physician to the facility are engaged in fee splitting which is unethical. (II)

6.06   **FEES: GROUP PRACTICE.** The division of income among members of a group, practicing jointly or in a partnership, may be determined by the members of the group and may be based on the value of the professional medical services performed by the member and his other services and contributions to the group. (II)

6.07   **INSURANCE FORM COMPLETION CHARGES.** The attending physician should complete without charge the appropriate "simplified" insurance claim form as a partof his service to the patient to enable the patient to receive his benefits. A charge for more complex forms may be made in comformity with local custom. (II)

6.08   **INTEREST CHARGES AND FINANCE CHARGES.** Although harsh or commercial collection practices are discouraged in the practice of medicine, a physician who has experienced problems with delinquent accounts may properly choose to request that payment be made at the time of treatment or add interest or other reasonable charges to delinquent accounts. The patient must be notified in advance of the interest or other reasonable finance or service charges by such means as the posting of a notice in the physician's waiting room, the distribution of leaflets describing the office billing practices and appropriate notations on the billing statement. The physician must comply with state and federal laws and regulations applicable to the imposition of such charges. The Council on Ethical and Judicial Affairs encourages physicians who choose to add an interest or finance charge to accounts not paid within a reasonable time to make exceptions in hardship cases. (II)

6.09   **LABORATORY BILL.** When it is not possible for the laboratory bill to be sent directly to the patient, the referring physician's bill to the patient should indicate the actual charges for laboratory services, including the name of the laboratory, as well as any separate charges for his own professional services. (II)

6.10   **SURGICAL ASSISTANT'S FEE.** Each physician engaged in the care of the patient is entitled to compensation commensurate with the value of the service he has personally rendered.

No physician should bill or be paid for a service which he does not perform; mere referral does not constitute a professional service for which a professional charge should be made or for which a fee may be ethically paid or received.

When services are provided by more than one physician, each physician should submit his own bill to the patient and be compensated separately, if possible.

It is ethically permissible in certain circumstances, however, for a surgeon to engage other physicians to assist him in the performance of a surgical procedure and to pay a reasonable amount for such assistance, provided the nature of the financial arrangement is made known to the patient. This principle applies whether or not the assisting physician is the referring physician. (II)

6.11   **COMPETITION.** Competition between and among physicians and other health care practitioners on the basis of competitive factors such as quality of services, skill, experience, miscellaneous conveniences offered to patients, credit terms, fees charged, etc., is not only ethical but is encouraged. Ethical medical practice thrives best under free market conditions when prospective patients have adequate information and opportunity to choose freely between and among competing physicians and alternate systems of medical care. (VII)

6.12   **FEES FOR MEDICAL SERVICES.** A physician should not charge or collect an illegal or excessive fee. For example, an illegal fee occurs when a physician accepts an assignment as full payment for services rendered to a Medicare patient and then bills the patient for an additional amount. A fee is excessive when after a review of the facts a person knowledgeable as to current charges made by physicians would be left with a definite and firm conviction that the fee is in excess of a reasonable fee. Factors to be considered as guides in determining the reasonableness of a fee include the following:

   A. the difficulty and/or uniqueness of the services performed and the time, skill and experience required;
   B. the fee customarily charged in the locality for similar physician services;
   C. the amount of the charges involved;
   D. the quality of performance;
   E. the nature and length of the professional relationship with the patient; and
   F. the experience, reputation and ability of the physician in performing the kind of services involved. (II)

7.00   OPINIONS ON PHYSICIAN RECORDS

7.01   RECORDS OF PHYSICIANS: AVAILABILITY OF INFORMATION TO OTHER PHYSICIANS. The interest of the patient is paramount in the practice of medicine, and everything that can reasonably and lawfully be done to serve that interest must be done by all physicians who have served or are serving the patient. A physician who formerly treated a patient should not refuse for any reason to make his records of that patient promptly available on request to another physician presently treating the patient. Proper authorization for the use of records must be granted by the patient. Medical reports should not be withheld because of an unpaid bill for medical services. (IV)

7.02   RECORDS OF PHYSICIANS: INFORMATION AND PATIENTS. Notes made in treating a patient are primarily for the physician's own use and constitute his personal property. However, on request of the patient a physician should provide a copy or a summary of the record to the patient or to another physician, an attorney, or other person designated by the patient.

Several states have enacted statutes that authorize patient access to medical records. These statutes vary in scope and mechanism for permitting patients to review or copy medical records. Access to mental health records, particularly, may be limited by statute or regulation. A physician should become familiar with the applicable laws, rules or regulations on patient access to medical records.

The record is a confidential document involving the physician-patient relationship and should not be communicated to a third party without the patient's prior written consent, unless required by law or to protect the welfare of the individual or the community. Medical reports should not be withheld because of an unpaid bill for medical services. Simplified, routine insurance reimbursement forms should be prepared without charge, but a charge for complex, complicated or multiple reports may be made in conformity with local custom. (IV)

7.03   RECORDS OF PHYSICIANS ON RETIREMENT. A patient's records may be necessary to the patient in the future not only for medical care but also for employment, insurance, litigation, or other reason. When a physician retires or dies, patients should be notified and urged to find a new physician and should be informed that upon authorization records will be sent to the new physician. Records which may be of value to a patient and which are not forwarded to a new physician should be retained, either by the physician himself, another

physician, or such other person lawfully permitted to act as a custodian of
the records. (IV)

7.04   **SALE OF A MEDICAL PRACTICE.** A physician or the estate of a deceased physician
may sell to another physician the elements which comprise his practice, such
as furniture, fixtures, equipment, office leasehold and goodwill. In the sale of
a medical practice, the purchaser is buying not only furniture and fixtures,
but also goodwill, i.e., the opportunity to take over the patients of the seller.
     The transfer of records of patients is subject, however, to the following:

1. All active patients should be notified that the physician (or his
    estate) is transferring the practice to another physician who will
    retain custody of their records and that at their written request,
    within a reasonable time as specified in the notice, the records or
    copies will be sent to any other physician of their choice. Rather
    than destroy the records of a deceased physician, it is better that they
    be transferred to a practicing physician who will retain them subject
    to requests from patients that they be sent to another physician.

2. A reasonable charge may be made for the cost of duplicating
    records. (IV)

8.00   OPINIONS ON PRACTICE MATTERS

8.01   APPOINTMENT CHARGES. A physician may charge a patient for a missed appointment or for one not cancelled 24 hours in advance if the patient is fully advised that the physician will make such a charge. The practice, however, should be resorted to infrequently and always with the utmost consideration for the patient and his circumstances. (VI)

8.02   CLINICS. Physicians practicing in a group or clinic are, both individually, and as a group, subject to the Principles of Medical Ethics. (VI)

8.03   CONFLICTS OF INTEREST: GUIDELINES. Physician ownership interest in a commercial venture with the potential for abuse is not in itself unethical. Physicians are free to enter lawful contractual relationships, including the acquisition of ownership interests in health facilities or equipment or pharmaceuticals. However, the potential conflict of interest must be addressed by the following: (1) the physician has an affirmative ethical obligation to disclose to the patient or referring colleagues his or her ownership interest in the facility or therapy prior to utilization; (2) the physician may not exploit the patient in any way, as by inappropriate or unnecessary utilization; (3) the physician's activities must be in strict conformance with the law; (4) the patient should have free choice either to use the physician's proprietary facility or therapy or to seek the needed medical services elsewhere; and (5) when a physician's commercial interest conflicts so greatly with the patient's interest as to be incompatible, the physician should make alternative arrangements for the care of the patient. (II,III,IV)

8.04   CONSULTATION. Physicians should obtain consultation whenever they believe that it would be helpful in the care of the patient or when requested by the patient or the patient's representative. When a patient is referred to a consultant, the referring physician should provide a history of the case and such other information as the consultant may need and the consultant should advise the referring physician of the results of the consultant's examination and recommendations relating to the management of the case. A physician selected by a patient for the purpose of obtaining a second opinion on an elective procedure is not obligated to advise the patient's regular physician of the findings or recommendations. (V)

8.05   **CONTRACTUAL RELATIONSHIPS.** The contractual relationships that physicians assume when they enter prepaid group practice plans are varied.

Income arrangements may include hourly wages for physicians working part time, annual salaries for those working full time, and share of group income for physicians who are partners in groups that are somewhat autonomous and contract with plans to provide the required medical care. Arrangements also usually include a range of fringe benefits, such as paid vacations, insurance and pension plans.

Physicians may work directly for plans or may be employed by the medical group or the hospital that has contracted with the plan to provide services. The AMA recognizes that under proper legal authority such plans may be established and that a physician may be employed by, or otherwise serve, a medical care plan. In the operation of such plans, physicians should not be subjected to lay interference in professional medical matters and their primary responsibility should be to the patients they serve. (VI)

8.06   **DRUGS AND DEVICES: PRESCRIBING.**

(1) A physician should not be influenced in the prescribing of drugs, devices or appliances by a direct or indirect financial interest in a pharmaceutical firm or other supplier. Whether the firm is a manufacturer, distributor, wholesaler or repackager of the products involved is immaterial.

(2) A physician may own or operate a pharmacy or dispense drugs if there is no resulting exploitation of patients.

(3) A physician should not give patients prescriptions in code or enter into agreements with pharmacies or other suppliers regarding the filling of prescriptions by code.

(4) Patients are entitled to the same freedom of choice in selecting who will fill their prescription needs as they are in the choice of a physician. (See 9.06 and 8.03.) The prescription is a written direction for a therapeutic or corrective agent. A patient is entitled to a copy of the physician's prescription for drugs, eyeglasses, contact lenses, or other devices as required by the Principles of Medical Ethics and as required by law. The patient has the right to have the prescription filled wherever the patient wishes.

(5) Patients have an ethically and legally recognized right to prompt access to the information contained in their individual medical records. The prescription is an essential part of the patient's medical record. Physicians should not discourage patients from requesting a written prescription or urge them to fill prescriptions from an establishment which has a direct telephone line or which has entered into a business or other preferential arrangement with the physician with respect to the filling of the physician's prescriptions. (I,II,III,IV,V)

8.07   HEALTH FACILITY OWNERSHIP BY A PHYSICIAN. A physician may own or have a financial interest in a for-profit hospital, nursing home or other health facility, such as a free-standing surgical center or emergency clinic. However, the physician has an affirmative ethical obligation to disclose his ownership of a health facility to his patient, prior to admission or utilization.

Under no circumstances may the physician place his own financial interest above the welfare of his patients. The prime objective of the medical profession is to render service to humanity; reward or financial gain is a subordinate consideration. For a physician to unnecessarily hospitalize a patient or prolong a patient's stay in the health facility for the physician's financial benefit would be unethical.

If a conflict develops between the physician's financial interest and the physician's responsibilities to the patient, the conflict must be resolved to the patient's benefit. (II)

8.08   INFORMED CONSENT. The patient's right of self-decision can be effectively exercised only if the patient possesses enough information to enable an intelligent choice. The patient should make his own determination on treatment. The physician's obligation is to present the medical facts accurately to the patient or to the individual responsible for his care and to make recommendations for management in accordance with good medical practice. The physician has an ethical obligation to help the patient make choices from among the therapeutic alternatives consistent with good medical practice. Informed consent is a basic social policy for which exceptions are permitted (1) where the patient is unconscious or otherwise incapable of consenting and harm from failure to treat is imminent; or (2) when risk-disclosure poses such a serious psychological threat of detriment to the patient as to be medically contraindicated. Social policy does not accept the paternalistic view that the physician may remain silent because divulgence might prompt the patient to forego needed therapy. Rational, informed patients should not be expected to act uniformly, even under similar circumstances, in agreeing to or refusing treatment. (I,II, III,IV,V)

8.09   LABORATORY SERVICES.

(1) A physician should not misrepresent or aid in the misrepresentation of laboratory services performed and supervised by a nonphysician as the physician's professional services. Such situations could involve a laboratory owned by a physician who directs and manages its financial and business affairs with no professional medical services being provided; laboratory work being performed by technicians and directly supervised by a medical technologist with no participation by the physician; or the physician's name being used in connection with the laboratory so as to create the appearance that it is owned, operated, and supervised by a physician when this is not so.

(2) If a laboratory is owned, operated, and supervised by a non-physician in accordance with state law and performs tests exclusively for physicians who receive the results and make their own medical interpretations, the following considerations would apply:

The physician's ethical responsibility is to provide his patients with high quality services. This includes services which he performs personally and those which he delegates to others. A physician should not utilize the services of any laboratory, irrespective of whether it is operated by a physician or non-physician, unless he has the utmost confidence in the quality of its services. He must always assume personal responsibility for the best interests of his patients. Medical judgment based upon inferior laboratory work is likewise inferior. Medical considerations, not cost, must be paramount when the physician chooses a laboratory. The physician who disregards quality as the primary criterion or who chooses a laboratory solely because it provides him with low cost laboratory services on which he charges the patient a profit, is not acting in the best interests of his patient. However, if reliable, quality laboratory services are available at lower cost, the patient should have the benefit of the savings. As a professional, the physician is entitled to fair compensation for his services. A physician should not charge a markup, commission, or profit on the services rendered by others. A physician should not charge for services that are not provided. A markup is an excessive charge that exploits patients if it is nothing more than a tacked on amount for a service already provided and accounted for by the laboratory. A physician may make an acquisition charge or processing charge. The patient should be notified of any such charge in advance. (I,II,III,IV,V)

8.10 **LIEN LAWS.** In states where there are lien laws, a physician may file a lien as a means of assuring payment of his fee provided his fee is fixed in amount and not contingent on the amount of settlement of the patient's claim against a third party. (I,VI)

8.11 **NEGLECT OF PATIENT.** Physicians are free to choose whom they will serve. The physician should, however, respond to the best of his ability in cases of emergency where first aid treatment is essential. Once having undertaken a case, the physician should not neglect the patient, nor withdraw from the case without giving notice to the patient, the relatives, or responsible friends sufficiently long in advance of withdrawal to permit another medical attendant to be secured. (I,VI)

8.12 **PATIENT INFORMATION.** The physician must properly inform the patient of the diagnosis and of the nature and purpose of the treatment undertaken or prescribed. The physician may not refuse to so inform the patient.(I,V)

8.13 **REFERRAL OF PATIENTS-DISCLOSURE OF LIMITATIONS.** When a physician agrees to provide treatment, he thereby enters into a contractual relationship and assumes an ethical obligation to treat the patient to the best of his ability. PPO and HMO contracts generally restrict the participating physician's scope of referral to medical specialists, diagnostic laboratories, and hospitals that have contractual arrangements with the PPO and HMO. Some plans also restrict the circumstances under which referrals may be made to contracting medical specialists. If the PPO or HMO does not permit referral to a noncontracting medical specialist or to a diagnostic or treatment facility when the physician believes that the patient's condition requires such services, the physician should so inform the patient so that the patient may decide whether to accept the outside referral at his own expense or confine himself to services available within the PPO or HMO. In determining whether treatment or diagnosis requires referral to outside specialty services, the physician should be guided by standards of good medical practice. (II,VI)

8.14 **SEXUAL MISCONDUCT IN THE PRACTICE OF MEDICINE.** Sexual misconduct in the practice of medicine violates the trust the patient reposes in the physician and is unethical. (I,II,IV)

8.15 **SUBSTANCE ABUSE.** It is unethical for a physician to practice medicine while under the influence of a controlled substance, alcohol, or other chemical agents which impair his ability to practice medicine. (I)

8.16 **SUBSTITUTION OF SURGEON WITHOUT PATIENT'S KNOWLEDGE OR CONSENT.** A surgeon who allows a substitute to operate on his patient without the patient's knowledge and consent is deceitful. The patient is entitled to choose his own physician and he should be permitted to acquiesce in or refuse to accept the substitution.

The surgeon's obligation to the patient requires him to perform the surgical operation: (1) within the scope of authority granted by the consent to the operation; (2) in accordance with the terms of the contractual relationship; (3) with complete disclosure of facts relevant to the need and the performance of the operation; and (4) utilizing his best skill.

It should be noted that it is the operating surgeon to whom the patient grants consent to perform the operation. The patient is entitled to the services of the particular surgeon with whom he or she contracts. The operating surgeon, in accepting the patient, is obligated to utilize his personal talents in the performance of the operation to the extent required by the agreement creating the physician-patient relationship. He cannot properly delegate to another the duties which he is required to perform personally.

Under the normal and customary arrangement with patients, and with reference to the usual form of consent to operation, the operating surgeon is obligated to perform the operation but may be assisted by residents or other surgeons. With the consent of the patient, it is not unethical for the operating surgeon to delegate the performance of certain aspects of the operation to his assistant provided this is done under his participatory supervision, i.e., he must scrub. If a resident or other physician is to perform the operation under non-participatory supervision, it is necessary to make a full disclosure of this fact to the patient, and this should be evidenced by an appropriate statement contained in the consent. Under these circumstances, it is the resident or other physician who becomes the operating surgeon. (I,II,IV,V)

9.00 OPINIONS ON PROFESSIONAL RIGHTS AND RESPONSIBILITIES

9.01 **ACCREDITATION.** Physicians who engage in activities that involve the accreditation, approval or certification of institutions, facilities and programs that provide patient care or medical education or certify the attainment of specialized professional competence have the ethical responsibility to apply standards that are relevant, fair, reasonable and nondiscriminatory. The accreditation of institutions and facilities that provide patient care should be based upon standards that focus upon the quality of patient care achieved. Standards used in the accreditation of patient care and medical education, or the certification of specialized professional attainment should not be adopted or used as a means of economic regulation. (II,IV,VII)

9.02 **AGREEMENTS RESTRICTING THE PRACTICE OF MEDICINE.** The Council on Ethical and Judicial Affairs discourages any agreement between physicians which restricts the right of a physician to practice medicine for a specified period of time or in a specified area upon termination of employment or a partnership or a corporate agreement. Such **restr**ictive agreements are not in the public interest. (VI,VII)

9.03 **CIVIL RIGHTS AND PROFESSIONAL RESPONSIBILITY.** The American Medical Association is in favor of equality of opportunity in medical society activities, medical education and training, employment, and all other aspects of medical professional endeavors regardless of race, color, religion, creed, ethnic affiliation, national origin, sex, age or handicap.

The American Medical Association is unalterably opposed to the denial of membership privileges and responsibilities in county medical societies and state medical associations to any duly licensed physician because of race, color, religion, creed, ethnic affiliation, national origin, sex, age or handicap. (IV)

9.04 **DISCIPLINE AND MEDICINE.** Incompetence, corruption or dishonest or unethical conduct on the part of members of the medical profession is reprehensible. In addition to posing a real or potential threat to patients, such conduct undermines the public's confidence in the profession. A physician should expose, without fear or favor, incompetent or corrupt, dishonest or unethical conduct on the part of members of the profession. Questions of such conduct should be considered, first, before proper medical tribunals in executive sessions or by special or duly appointed committees on ethical relations, provided such a course is possible and provided, also, that the law is not hampered thereby. If doubt should arise as to the legality of the physician's conduct, the situation under investigation should be placed before officers of the law, and the physician-investigators should take the necessary steps to enlist the interest of the proper authority.

An ethical physician will observe the laws regulating the practice of medicine and will not assist others to evade such laws.

The Council cannot pass judgment in advance on a situation that may later come before it on appeal. The Council cannot be an attorney for a society or a member thereof and later judge in the same factual situation. The local medical society has the initial obligation of determining all the facts and whether or not disciplinary action is indicated. Questions asking for a review of a proposed course of action or an evaluation of an existing factual situation should be presented to the appropriate official of the physician's local society. (II,III,VII)

9.05   **DUE PROCESS.** The basic principles of a fair and objective hearing should always be accorded to the physician whose professional conduct is being reviewed. The fundamental aspects of a fair hearing are: a listing of specific charges, adequate notice of the right of a hearing, the opportunity to be present and to rebut the evidence, and the opportunity to present a defense. These principles apply when the hearing body is a medical society tribunal or a hospital committee composed of physicians.

These principles of fair play apply in all disciplinary hearings and in any other type of hearing in which the physician may be deprived of valuable property rights. Whenever physicians sit in judgment on physicians and whenever that judgment affects a physician's reputation, professional status, or livelihood, these principles of fair play must be observed.

All physicians are urged to observe diligently these fundamental safeguards of due process whenever they are called upon to serve on a committee which will pass judgment on physicians. Medical societies and hospital medical staffs are urged to review the constitution and bylaws of the society or hospital medical staff to make sure that these instruments provide for such procedural safeguards. (II,III,VII)

9.06   **FREE CHOICE.** Free choice of physicians is the right of every individual. One may select and change at will one's physicians, or one may choose a medical care plan such as that provided by a closed panel or group practice or health maintenance or service organization. The individual's freedom to select a preferred system of health care and free competition among physicians and alternative systems of care are prerequisites of ethical practice and optimal patient care.

In choosing to subscribe to a health maintenance or service organization or in choosing or accepting treatment in a particular hospital, the patient is thereby accepting limitations upon free choice of medical services.

The need of an individual for emergency treatment in cases of accident or sudden illness may, as a practical matter, preclude free choice of physician, particularly where there is loss of consciousness.

Although the concept of free choice assures that an individual can generally choose a physician, likewise a physician may decline to accept that individual as a patient. In selecting the physician of choice, the patient may sometimes be obliged to pay for medical services which might otherwise be paid by a third party. (IV)

9.07   MEDICAL TESTIMONY. As a citizen and as a professional with special training and experience, the physician has an ethical obligation to assist in the administration of justice. If a patient who has a legal claim requests his physician's assistance, the physician should furnish medical evidence, with the patient's consent, in order to secure the patient's legal rights.

The medical witness must not become an advocate or a partisan in the legal proceeding. The medical witness should be adequately prepared and should testify honestly and truthfully. The attorney for the party who calls the physician as a witness should be informed of all favorable and unfavorable information developed by the physician's evaluation of the case. It is unethical for a physician to accept compensation that is contingent upon the outcome of litigation. (II,IV,V,VII)

9.08   NEW MEDICAL PROCEDURES. In the ethical tradition expressed by Hippocrates and continuously affirmed thereafter, the role of the physician has been that of a healer who serves patients, a teacher who imparts knowledge of skills and techniques to colleagues, and a student who constantly seeks to keep abreast of new medical knowledge.

Physicians have an obligation to share their knowledge and skills and to report the results of clinical and laboratory research. This tradition enhances patient care, leads to the early evaluation of new technologies, and permits the rapid dissemination of improved techniques.

The intentional withholding of new medical knowledge, skills, and techniques from colleagues for reasons of personal gain is detrimental to the medical profession and to society and is to be condemned.

Prompt presentation before scientific organizations and timely publication of clinical and laboratory research in scientific journals are essential elements in the foundation of good medical care. (I,II,V,VII)

9.09 **PATENT FOR SURGICAL OR DIAGNOSTIC INSTRUMENT.** A physician may patent a surgical or diagnostic instrument he has discovered or developed. The laws governing patents are based on the sound doctrine that one is entitled to protect his discovery. (V,VII)

9.10 **PEER REVIEW.** Medical society ethics committees, hospital credentials and utilization committees, and other forms of peer review have been long established by organized medicine to scrutinize physicians' professional conduct. At least to some extent, each of these types of peer review can be said to impinge upon the absolute professional freedom of physicians. They are, nonetheless, recognized and accepted. They are necessary. They balance the physician's right to exercise his medical judgment freely with his obligation to do so wisely and temperately. (II,III,VII)

9.11 **PHYSICIAN IMPAIRMENT.** In order to protect patients and the public, physicians have the responsibility to report to the appropriate body credible evidence of a colleague's impairment that may affect competence. Such impairment may result from abuse of drugs or alcohol, or from mental or physical illness. All physicians have an obligation to urge impaired colleagues to seek treatment. (II)

9.12 **PHYSICIAN-PATIENT RELATIONSHIP: RESPECT FOR LAW AND HUMAN RIGHTS.** The creation of the physician-patient relationship is contractual in nature. Generally, both the physician and the patient are free to enter into or decline the relationship. A physician may decline to undertake the care of a patient whose medical condition is not within the physician's current competence. However, physicians who offer their services to the public may not decline to accept patients because of race, color, religion, national origin, or any other basis that would constitute illegal discrimination. Furthermore, physicians who are obligated under preexisting contractual arrangements may not decline to accept patients as provided by those arrangements. (I,III,V,VI)

9.13 **PHYSICIANS AND INFECTIOUS DISEASES.** A physician who knows that he or she has an infectious disease, which if contracted by the patient would pose a significant risk to the patient, should not engage in any activity that creates a risk of transmission of that disease to the patient. The precautions taken to prevent the transmission of a contagious disease to a patient should be appropriate to the seriousness of the disease and must be particularly stringent in the case of a disease that is potentially fatal. (I,IV)

INDEX

APPENDIX B

Hippocratic Oath

The Hippocratic Oath is the physician's oath of conduct that provides guidelines for conduct with patient relations and treatment.

Many healthcare consumers have heard references to the Hippocratic Oath. Very few have had the opportunity to read it.

The oath obligates a doctor to certain relationship with other doctors, their families, their patients and their lives.

HIPPOCRATIC OATH

Unabridged and as published in 1943

I swear by Apollo Physician, by Asclepius, by Health, by Heal-All, and by all the gods and goddesses, that, according to my ability and judgment, I will keep this oath and stipulation; to reckon him who taught me this art equally dear to me as my parents, and share my substance with him and relieve his necessities if required. To regard his offspring as on the same footing with my own brothers and to teach them this art if they should wish to learn it, without fee or stipulation; and that by precept, lecture and every other mode of instruction I will impart a knowledge of the art to my own sons and to those of my teachers and to disciples bound by a stipulation and oath, according to the law of medicine, but to none others.

I will follow that method of treatment which, according to my ability and judgment, I consider for the benefit of my patients, and abstain from whatever is deleterious and mischievous. I will give no deadly medicine to anyone if asked, nor suggest any such counsel. Furthermore, I will not give to a woman an instrument to produce an abortion.

With Purity and with Holiness I will pass my life and practice my art. I will not cut a person who is suffering with a stone, but will leave this to be done by practitioners of this work. Into whatever houses I enter I will go into them for the benefit of the sick and will abstain from every voluntary act of mischief and corruption; and further from the seduction of females or males, bond or free.

Whatever, in connection with my professional practice, or not in connection with it, I may see or hear in the lives of men which ought not to be spoken abroad, I will not divulge, as reckoning that all such should be kept secret.

While I continue to keep this oath unviolated, may it be granted to me to enjoy life and the practice of the art, respected by all men, at all times, but should I trespass and violate this oath, may the reverse be my lot.

INDEX

Ten Top Reasons Not To Go To The Hospital:

10.   Luxury resorts are less expensive.

9.   Food and service is better at luxury resorts.

8.   It is unnecessary for 40% of the patients.

7.   10% of all patients get a hospital acquired infection.

6.   It is where doctors get their practice (on-the-job-training).
     (In any other business, interns and residents would be called "management trainees.")

5.   There is a 3 to 4% chance of receiving the wrong medication.

4.   It may not fix your problem.

3.   No warranties are provided.

2.   There is a 1 in 10 chance that you will be readmitted.

1.   It hurts; physically, emotionally and financially!

If your healthcare provider recommends hospitalization, by all means go; after you are absolutely certain of your healthcare provider's qualifications and necessity of treatment.

QUALITY

Quality — (Kwôl'itē) N., the **degree of excellence** a thing possesses.

Quality control — A system of maintaining **desired standards** of a product or process.

What are the **desired standards** by which America measures the **degree of excellence** of healthcare?

> Was the healthcare provider friendly?*
> Was the healthcare provider attentive?*
> Was the healthcare provider accessible?*

*NOTE: *"Healthcare quality good"* was the headline for actual survey results that used these standards to judge the quality of U.S. healthcare. By these standards the United States probably does have the often quoted statement; "The highest quality healthcare in the world."

If these same standards were applied to United States auto manufacturers, they would not have their current problems with imports.

LIGHT JOKES

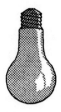

Question: How many **chiropractors** does it take to change a light bulb?

Answer: One, but it takes 33 visits.

Question: How many **psychiatrists** does it take to change a light bulb?

Answer: One, but the light bulb has to want to change.

Question: How many **cardiologists** does it take to change a light bulb?

Answer: One, but they only hold the light bulb, the world revolves around them.

HEALTHCARE MYTHS

1) **Patients aren't smart enough to understand.**

   * Not true. Talk to anyone who has undergone extensive medical treatment and they can talk the medical lingo as well as any medical provider.

2) **Patient doesn't want to know.**

   * Not true. Some don't, but most do want to know so that they can become an active participant in their treatment.

3) **Patient can't refuse doctor's orders.**

   * Not true. This is done every day when patients do not follow the doctor's orders to take drugs as prescribed. The patient can always refuse doctor's orders. The patient is in control.

4) **Doctors are Gods.**

   * Not true. They are only Gods if the patient allows them to be. A doctor's spouse, friends, peers and subordinates probably would confirm that they definitely are not Gods.

5) **United States has the best healthcare in the world.**

   * Not true. Only when measured by cost and tools available. When measured by life expectancy, infant mortality, population's accessibility to medical care and other such indicators, it is below the rest of the industrialized world.

6) **National healthcare will solve all our problems.**

   * Not true. All it will do is reward the healthcare providers for their excess capacity.

AN UNSCIENTIFIC OPINION POLL

This opinion poll makes no effort to follow industry standard scientific polling methods and statistical analysis. It is done to demonstrate that results may be different if more choices are provided.

The question is:

If you were stranded on a desert island, which of the following would you take with you to relieve your pain and suffering?

☐ Aspirin   ☐ Tylenol™

☐ Bufferin™   ☐ Advil™

☐ Anacin™   ☐ An attractive member
                               of the human species

HELP WANTED

EARN 5 times the U.S. average income.

Enjoy — 60% profit margins
— Limited competition
— High community prestige

Full Benefit Package:

* Luxury car and all expenses
* Free trips (room, meals and entertainment included)
  — Need to attend two hour educational meeting
* Free or discounted office space
* Free or discounted loans
* 25% contribution to retirement plan

Other Benefits:

1) You can say "trust me" and the customer will believe you.
2) **Be nice** and the customer will think you provide **high quality care**.
3) Customer doesn't ask about price.
4) You can **increase prices**, even when faced with competition.
5) Customers are willing to wait one hour for 3 to 4 minutes of your services.
6) Increase sales by referring customers to your other companies without fear of "conflict of interest" accusations.

Requirements: Speak foreign language (medical jargon)
Seven years of college
Three years as "management trainee"

Send resume to: Box IAMADR
Medical Towers
Beverly Hills, CA 90210

AN UNSCIENTIFIC OPINION POLL II

This opinion poll makes no effort to follow industry standard scientific polling methods and statistical analysis. It is done to demonstrate that results may be different if more choices are provided.

The question is:

What percent (%) of a doctor's gross income is spent for medical malpractice insurance?

	0-10%	10-20%	20-30%	30-40%	40%+
All Doctors	☐	☐	☐	☐	☐

BUY THIS BOOK FOR
A FRIEND OR LOVED ONE

Just send your name, address and a check or money order for $19.95 (plus $3.00 postage and handling) to:

Med. Ed.
P.O. Box 40696
Mesa, AZ 85274

Makes a great gift!

Enclosed is $19.95 (plus $3.00 shipping and handling, mailed 4th Class or $5.00 shipping and handling for 1st Class mailing) in check or money order, payable to Med. Ed. Inc. (Arizona add 6% tax).

Name _____

Address _____

City/State/Zip _____

Med. Ed. ● P.O. Box 40696
Mesa, AZ 85274

Enclosed is $19.95 (plus $3.00 shipping and handling, mailed 4th Class or $5.00 shipping and handling for 1st Class mailing) in check or money order, payable to Med. Ed. Inc. (Arizona add 6% tax).

Name _____

Address _____

City/State/Zip _____

Med. Ed. ● P.O. Box 40696
Mesa, AZ 85274